THE MENOPAUSE SURVIVAL GUIDE

Surviving the Change of Life

Donna Rogers

Oakview Press
Kansas City, Missouri

THE MENOPAUSE SURVIVAL GUIDE
Surviving the Change of Life
Donna Rogers
Published by:
Oakview Press
P.O.Box 28114
Kansas City, MO 64188-0114 U.S.A.
OakviewPress@aol.com
www.MenopauseSurvivalGuide.com

Unattributed quotations are by Donna Rogers.

ISBN 0-9725348-0-6

First printing 2002

Printed in the United States of America

Library of Congress Data

Rogers, Donna
The Menopause Survival Guide :
Surviving the Change of Life
First edition
Includes index
ISBN 0-9725348-0-6
Library of Congress Control Number: 2002094982

TABLE OF CONTENTS

WARNING - DISCLAIMER

The purpose of the *Menopause Survival Guide* is to provide basic information about most of the issues associated with menopause. It is not meant to be a definitive source, but a composite of generally known information that can be referenced quickly and understood easily. In no way is the *Menopause Survival Guide* meant to replace the medical advice of your physician. Before engaging in any exercise program, diet, or medication treatment (either non-prescription or prescription), you should consult your physician.

In the same way that your physician may suggest you secure a second opinion, it is recommended that you do your own additional research about menopause. An abbreviated list of websites is available on page 150. This is not a comprehensive list of sources, but it is a good starting place. Your public library and the internet abound with information. Be a discerning reader and purchaser.

Dedication

To my family (especially Alan) who has always shown me love, supported me in tough times, encouraged me in my endeavors, cared for me when I was ill, laughed with me in good times, shared my dreams, and has never, even once, failed to be there for me.

And to my Reunion Group friends. You are the best girlfriends in the world! Life is better with you in it.

I Love You All!

Thank you for reading my book.

I hope it helps you understand your body a little better, inspires you to learn even more, and brings a spot of humor into your day.

Let's get started...........

1
Menopause and Me

Hello Reader.....

Before we get started, let's get acquainted. My name is Donna Rogers. I was born in 1951 in St. Joseph, Missouri and share a birthday with Charlie Brown (although he's a year older.) The DeShon family moved to Kansas City when I was three, and we've lived here ever since. I'm a graduate of North Kansas City High School and still visit with about 20 of my fellow Hornet girlfriends once a month. In 1973 I graduated from Missouri Western College with a degree in English and Education, and in 1976 I married Alan Rogers, my wonderful husband and friend. (We don't have any kids.) I have been blessed with a great family and friends.

My life was never eventful enough to make the talk shows, but it's been interesting. For example, Alan was already a radio announcer when we married, so he encouraged me to get my license, and together we had a Christian radio ministry for several years. And I've taught a variety of classes through our local adult education programs. But mostly, I've been quite content being a housewife, pursuing my hobbies, and enjoying my loved ones. I think everyone entertains the idea of writing a book or a song, but I never intended to make that a reality and actually become an author. But here I am. WHY? Because of menopause.

Menopause is the weirdest thing I've ever encountered. When I first became "menopausal," I knew little more than that my periods were becoming irregular. Then the hot flashes started, followed by the waves of uncontrolled moodiness and tears. It was time to learn more about menopause.

I have always kept track of my periods, so on my yearly visits to the gynecologist, he was able to quickly confirm that my periods were changing and that I was indeed entering menopause. He was willing to answer any questions, but I didn't know what to ask. He gave me a prescription for hormone replacement, some comments about the pros and cons of HRT, and permission to discontinue the pills if I didn't like how they affected my body.

I know some women love HRT, but I didn't. I got very sick with cramps and nearly became anemic. At the end of the three weeks, I had had enough and discontinued the pills. I've not taken any since. This is not a comment for or against HRT, only my own personal experience.

My next visit was to the woman who has always explained all these "girl" experiences. My mom. When I asked for her advice about how she went through menopause, Mom said that she never took HRT and got through it just fine; that the hot flashes and everything else were annoying, sometimes maddening, but that they pass. So, like mother/like daughter, I decided to go through this menopause thing cold turkey. It might not be right for everyone, but it worked best for me.

It seemed that no matter where I looked, there was an article or pamphlet on menopause. I read everything I could. Did research on the internet. Talked to women everywhere about how they were handling menopause. Unfortunately, what I found was a lot of information that didn't always agree. For every pro, there was a con. For every con, there was a pro. I learned surviving menopause is not a cut-and-dried matter.

Some of the information was in very technical terminology. I don't know about anyone else, but I just wasn't familiar with eye-popping terms like *oophorectomy, amenorrhea* or, my favorite, *the luteinizing hormone-releasing hormone.*

Other information was too simplified. For example, there are endless lists of the different ways estrogen affects the female body. But I wanted to know WHY losing estrogen will cause wrinkles. And I sure wanted to know WHY estrogen changes might make me grow facial hair. (yikes!)

Some information was just TOO depressing. The last thing I needed was a heavy psychological treatise on top of all the distressing stuff already happening to my body. On the contrary, it was soon apparent to me that a healthy dose of humor is essential in surviving menopause.

The best information is what I learned about the female body. We are a fascinating creation! I had never thought about it but wasn't surprised to learn that the hormones that affect menopausal women are the same ones that affect PMS sufferers and pregnant women. In fact, it's hard to talk about only menopause, in and of itself, because the entire menstrual process has affected women from puberty right on through the actual menopause.

So, that's why I've written the *Menopause Survival Guide*. I wanted to share with other women what I've learned about what menopause is, why it causes the symptoms it does, and what can be done to "survive" this weird time of life.

Since family members have to accompany you on this roller coaster ride, I've included a chapter called *Surviving the Change of Wife*, an easy-to-understand section for husbands. If you're married, be sure your honey reads it. There is also a special section for kids about surviving the change of mom. I call it *Meno Moms*.

I wanted to make this a concise, one-stop book about menopause. It's not meant to be a replacement for regular medical advice from your physician, but it can be a useful resource guide.

If even one woman is helped by reading my book, then I will consider it a success.

Blessings to you!

Donna Rogers

2
Women's Health
Finally......some open talk

Up until recently, menopause hasn't been a widely discussed issue. Life expectancies were so low that hardly any women lived long enough to get to the age of menopause! And even if they had, adverse living conditions would have prevented them from being aware of it. Most women were so occupied from sunup to sundown with chores and just staying alive that they didn't have much time to notice, let alone worry about, going through the Change.

Of course, medical care was nothing like it is today, and many women (and men) died far too young because of that.

Probably the advent of climate-controlled rooms (thanks to heating and air conditioning) and a well-pampered Western society are greatly responsible for making menopause a talked-about issue.

Ancient "Hysterical" Women

Of course, not all olden-times women died early. More than a few women must have lived to the age of menopause during the time of the ancient Greeks and Romans because it was ancient Greek men who came up with the word *hysterectomy.* They based it on their word *hysterical* leading us to assume that they were more than familiar with the wild mood swings of menopausal Greek women.

Modern Women

However, it wasn't until early in the 20th century when most women were actually living long enough to go through all the stages of menopause that much became known about it. Today, the average American woman lives to be around 80 years old, and she experiences the full spectrum of menopausal symptoms in all their glory. Yet, it's only been recently that the subject has been openly discussed. Prior to that, "nice" girls just didn't talk about such things!

The Mother/Daughter Talk

Many mothers were too shy to talk to their daughters about periods (and then sex) because their mothers before them had been too shy to talk about the same issues. Even if they did try to share what they knew, such subjects can be hard to explain, and even harder for a young mind to comprehend. Yet who was to explain menopause to the mom? Her mother was probably of the old school where they didn't talk about such delicate subjects. Even if a grandma had been open to talk about menopause, she probably didn't know much more than to say *You're going to stop having periods. Before that happens, you're going to have about 10 years when your periods come and go, and sometimes they'll be really heavy. You're also going to get cranky, sweaty at night, and hot during the day.* There was virtually no public education about menopause. It sure wasn't in all the magazines and on all the talk shows as it is today.

Consider the language formerly used to talk about women's issues. Periods were called *monthlies, that time of the month, the curse,* and ridiculous code names like *a visit from Aunt Flo* (flow). Being pregnant was *being in a family way* or *expecting a visit from the stork.* The initials *PG* might be whispered ever so discreetly. Menopause was, only, *The Change.*

At long last, women's issues are openly talked about. Even if we can't stop what's happening in our body, it does help to understand it. More importantly, open discussion is helping us to be healthier. Prior to this current time, most women did not see a gynecologist unless they were having a baby. Even in the 1980's, some people thought it was wrong for an unmarried female to go for a pap smear. That kind of backward thinking caused a lot of women (including teenage girls and unmarried women) to suffer needlessly with treatable disorders like painful cramps due to undiagnosed endometriosis or, worse, to die because of undiscovered cancers.

Bookstores, magazine articles, talk shows, and internet sites abound with information about PMS, menstrual periods, pap smears, and menopause. It is finally OK to talk about what's going on in our body.

There is so much to learn about menopause.

Only Three Types of Women Need To Know About Menopause:

Those Who Have Gone Through It,
Those Who Will Go Through It,
and
Those Who Are Going Through It Now!

3

Menopause

What It Is

MENOPAUSE

The word **MENOPAUSE** is derived from the Greek words *MENO* meaning *monthly,* and *PAUSIS* meaning *cessation.* In simple terms, a woman stops having a monthly period. And when has not had a period for one year, she has reached the medical definition of *menopause.* Menopause is also called the **Climacteric** which refers to the *climax* or *grand finale.* In a broad sense, climacteric means any crucial period in the life of a person. More specifically, it refers to the time of menopause, when fertility and sexuality start to decline. (*CLIMAX* comes from a word meaning *ladder.* Apparently, menopause was considered the last rung in the ladder of life.)

But menopause is much more than the single event of no longer having periods. For some women, that is the least of the menopausal process. Menopause truly is a Change of Life because we are permanently changed, physically and emotionally. Nearly everything seems to revolve around the changes menopause brings about. It is definitely a NEW experience.

Although it's no fun, menopause is a necessity and a blessing. Think about it. If our ovaries didn't shut down, we would remain fertile forever. That means we could get pregnant at 78. And you can take it to the bank that FEW women are interested in being 78 and pregnant. Not only that, without menopause, women would continue having periods right up until we die. What a gruesome thought!

Medical types often divide menopause into three stages. **Pre-menopause**, **menopause**, and **post-menopause**. That may be trying to split hairs because menopause is actually one big process, just with different manifestations. Most of the symptoms commonly associated with menopause occur during the pre-menopause, called **perimenopause.** This is when periods get irregular, mood swings are the wildest, and hot flashes and night sweats are the worst. Then about ten years later comes the actual **menopause** which is nothing more than an anniversary date of not having periods for one year. (Yippee!) The **post-menopause** is the rest of the woman's life, and is usually when the worst effects like osteoporosis or cancer may occur. Unless it is specifically defined, whenever the word MENOPAUSE is mentioned in the *Menopause Survival Guide*, it refers to the entire menopausal process.

PERIMENOPAUSE

Before we actually reach menopause, there is a 5-10 year transition period known as **perimenopause**. (*PERI* is a prefix meaning *near.*) This is the pre-menopausal phase which usually starts when a woman is in her 40's. It is the time when estrogen levels first begin to decline. The production of eggs slows, the hormone progesterone decreases, and the hormone estrogen fluctuates. It is during this peri-menopause that women will experience the symptoms most associated with menopause such as hot flashes, night sweats, vaginal dryness, loss of interest in sex, chest pain, shortness of breath, mood swings, memory difficulties, panic attacks, fatigue, irritability, and even depression. Physiological changes begin in peri-menopause that may develop into serious concerns later. For example, the bone loss that later causes osteoporosis occurs during the first seven years of perimenopause. Rises in cholesterol, increased blood pressure and weight gain may contribute to heart disease or stroke. And the loss of tissue strength may later cause uterine prolapse or bladder incontinence.

POST-MENOPAUSE

A woman's life seems to be divided into two halves: Before menopause and after menopause. The post-menopausal stage is everything that happens once periods officially stop. Most of the hot flashes and mood swings have settled down, but you may now be facing more serious complaints like those described in the above paragraph. Most women agree, however, that post-menopause is a cakewalk compared to the wild and crazy perimenopause years.

Because ovulation continues throughout peri-menopause, even though on an intermittent basis, a woman may become pregnant. Do not assume that just because you are entering menopause that you cannot become pregnant.

One Woman's Story

For years, we were the only caregiver for our elderly neighbors. It had been a long 17 years, and it was at its worst when the old gentleman had to be placed in a nursing home. Even the best nursing home is a terrible place. So many sweet people, so ill, so unable to take care of themselves, so alone. I made it a point to visit him every day, even though towards the end, he had no idea who I was.

In addition to many of the residents, I got to know two wonderful ladies who tirelessly planned activities and encouraged the patients. One was a widow, the other a nun. Both were in their 70's. While passing their office on one particularly emotionally draining day, they asked how I was doing. Unexpectedly, I found myself dissolving in tears. As we talked about the stress involved in being a caregiver, out of the clear blue, I told them that I was also in the middle of this stupid menopause thing. What happened next has left a lasting impression.

Both ladies smiled the knowing smile of someone who has been there. As we shared experiences, we were suddenly as one. The 30+ years difference in our ages disappeared. I don't know why, but when I saw reserved little Sister G giggling like a girl about hot flashes and crying jags, I realized that all women are made of the same stuff. Talk about a common bond!!!

4

Crazy Names For Operations and Hormones

Caution! Caution! Caution!

THE WEIRD WORDS ZONE

For some unknown reason, the medical community has chosen to give lengthy and unpronounceable names to most medical terms. This is probably because it was done by men. Most of this was done way back in the time of the ancient Greeks and Romans. Perhaps spouting fifty-dollar words made doctors feel important. Certainly using huge words made a doctor appear quite impressive and well-versed to his barely-educated patients. And if a doctor used a term that was totally unfamiliar to his patient, how could the patient possibly question the diagnosis or treatment mode when she didn't have a clue what the ol' doc was talking about? It's way too late to change all this medical lingo, but you can bet that if a woman could have done the naming, the terms would be much simpler. We'll look at a few examples.

Let's start with **hysterectomy.** The base word is *hysteric* which means *suffering in the womb.* (*Ectomy* means *to cut out.*) It is from the ancient Greek word for *hysterical* because they thought that women were hysterical more often than men. (Guess even Greek women had wild mood swings!) Had a woman named this operation, she would have cut to the chase and simply called it a **uterus removal**.

Frequently, when the uterus is removed, so are the ovaries. This surgery is called an **oophorectomy**. For such a serious surgery, it sure has a goofy name. Oophorectomy comes from the words meaning *egg + to bear + to cut out*. It literally means *cutting out the place that causes eggs to be born.* Hardly anyone in the world has heard of *OOPHORECTOMY*, although having this operation means the end of estrogen, egg production, and female fertility. That's pretty big stuff. More simple terms would be **ovary removal** or ovaries removal. UNILATERAL OOPHORECTOMY could more simply be called "one ovary removal." BILATERAL OOPHORECTOMY would be the "removal of both ovaries." By the way, the *oophor* part sounds like our phrase *two-fer.*

Hormones carry some $50 names, too. You will soon learn about the **Gonadotropin Hormones.** *Gonad* comes from a word meaning *to produce seed.* It refers to the seed-producing sex glands, which are the ovaries in women and testes in men. *Tropin* is a suffix that means *responds to a stimulus.* In real terms, these hormones would more easily be called **hormones to stimulate the ovaries**, or hormones to stimulate the testes (when referring to males.)

Speaking of gonads, look at the lovely **Gonadotropin Releasing Hormone-Antagonist (GnRH-antagonist.)** (How's that for a mouthful?) This rascal is a hormone that prevents the gonadotropin hormone from being released so that the ovaries aren't stimulated to produce estrogen. (whew) It would have been SO much simpler to call it what it is....An estrogen blocker!

And, finally, the medical community likes to use two different words for the same thing. The terms for the expanding of blood vessels are **Dilation** and **Dilatation**. Both mean the same thing. For some reason, someone along the way decided to throw in an extra syllable.

What you will find as you read is that most of the weird terms are pretty much just an explanation of the function or action of the hormone, operation, etc. There's no question, though, that the terminology surely would have been easier to understand had it been written in every-day real-person terms.

DON'T be overwhelmed when you start encountering these wild terms. You have to know them so you won't have a blank look on your face when the doctor starts discussing them. When these terms appear in the *Menopause Survival Guide*, every attempt has been made to explain them in plain language. You will also find a definition of terms in the Glossary at the back of this book.

Now, for the biggest terminology question:

If menopause is a woman's problem,
why does it start with MEN?

5

Women

The Workings of the Female Body

To best understand menopause, you have to understand the workings of the female body. Just like a car, we have all kinds of individual components that work together so that we are one smooth-running machine. However, also like a car, when even one of those components get out of whack, the car will cough, sputter, and maybe even break down. As menopause approaches, it is the coughing and sputtering of a hormone called **estrogen** that can make your body run not-so smoothly. Let's look at how these bodies of ours actually work.

FEMALE BODY

The word **hormone** comes from a Greek word meaning *to stimulate*. A hormone is a substance formed in some organ of the body and then carried by a body fluid to another organ or tissue on which it has a specific effect. Estrogen is one of several female sex hormones produced primarily by the ovaries and, in smaller amounts, by a hormone secreted by the adrenal gland that is converted into estrogen in the fat tissues of the body. Estrogen is kind of like an internal regulator that has an effect on nearly every part of our body.

ESTROGEN

Estrogen production starts inside the womb at around four and a half months. Because of estrogen (with a little help from progesterone) girls are born with an extra layer of fat. (This extra layer of fat is important for estrogen production, as you'll see later.) When it is time for puberty, estrogen first causes the "budding" of breasts, the rounding of hips and thighs, and the growth of pubic and underarm hair. About a year later, estrogen will cause the ovaries to mature, and monthly periods will begin. (A girl's first menstrual period is called the **menarche,** pronounced *men ARE key.*) The phase of puberty is considered complete when the girl's periods start to come on a regular basis.

At birth, females have about 1 million immature eggs in each ovary although, in the course of our lifetime, only about 200 per ovary will mature and be released during ovulation. Each ovary contains numerous cavities (sacs) called **follicles** in which the egg cells develop. Inside these follicles are small glands that secrete hormones such as estrogen and progesterone.

Also influencing hormone production is the **pituitary gland**, the body's master gland. The pituitary gland is a small, oval endocrine gland attached to the base of the brain. It secretes hormones influencing body growth, metabolism, and the activity of other endocrine glands. (An endocrine gland produces one or more chemicals (hormones) which go directly into the bloodstream where they are carried to other parts of the body. When they reach their destination, they regulate or control the functions of that body part.)

Directly connected to the pituitary gland is a part of the brain called the **hypothalamus.** Although it is only about the size of a marble, this brain region is the master control center for hormones. When the hypothalamus secretes hormone "messengers" to glands such as the pituitary, adrenal, and thyroid, these glands are stimulated to release their own hormones. Not surprising, the hormones from the hypothalamus are called hormone-releasing hormones.

HORMONES and the MENSTRUAL CYCLE

On the first day of a menstrual period, a woman's estrogen level is very low. The hypothalamus picks up these levels and sends a message to the pituitary gland via chemical messengers called **gonadotropin-releasing hormones (GnRH).** The pituitary gland releases the first set of its gonadotropin hormones, the **follicle stimulating hormones (FSH)**. These are designed to stimulate the follicles within the ovaries (gonads) so that they begin to grow. In fact, about 20 follicles will resume production of one of the forms of estrogen called **estradiol**. On day 5, the pituitary begins to gradually produce and release increasing amounts of the second of the gonadotropin hormones called the **luteinizing hormone (LH)**. Of the 20 or so follicles, only one will fully ripen. Between Days 12 and 14, with estrogen production at a peak, the pituitary gland sends an extra burst of LH which stimulates the follicle to burst and shoot out an egg.

While all this has been going on, estrogen has also caused the endometrium (uterine lining) to thicken to prepare the uterus for the possibility of fertilization. (This is called the **proliferative** or **follicular phase**. *Proliferative* means *promoting fertility. Follicular* refers to the development of an egg in the follicle.)

Once the egg is released, the empty follicle fills up with blood and forms a mass of yellow tissue called a **corpus luteum**. (This literally means *yellow body*.) As the follicles of the ovary continue to be stimulated through the second half of the menstrual cycle, in addition to continuing to produce estrogen, the corpus luteum within the ovary now also starts producing **progesterone**.

Progesterone is a steroid (sex) hormone that is active in preparing the uterus for the reception and development of the fertilized egg. The secretion of progesterone causes the delicate blood vessels of the uterine lining to swell up with blood. In the event of a pregnancy, this thick lining would nourish the fertilized egg. (This is called the **secretory** or **luteal phase** referring to the secretion of progesterone by the corpus luteum.)

The uterine lining is a network of **capillaries.** These incredibly tiny blood vessels have narrow diameters not much bigger than the blood cells flowing through them. The walls of capillaries are very thin and permeable. If an egg is fertilized, the permeability allows nutrients to pass from the mother's bloodstream into the developing egg. If an egg is not fertilized, the thinness of the walls allows them to burst so that the un-needed uterine lining can be shed. (Obviously, blood vessels literally exploding under pressure would not a good thing elsewhere in the body, but it's essential in the uterine department.)

Once the egg has been released and the uterine lining is nice and thick, two things happen. First, the high levels of progesterone and low levels of estrogen reach the hypothalamus and the pituitary which "tell" them to slow down the flow of the LH and FSH. Then, if the egg doesn't have a rendezvous with a sperm, the corpus luteum will dry up and stop sending out progesterone and estrogen. When the progesterone drops off sharply enough, the capillaries will burst, and the blood-swollen uterine lining, along with the unfertilized egg, will be expelled in what we know as menstruation. This usually happens about 14 days after the ovulation, and is considered Day 1 of the menstrual cycle.

HORMONES and PREGNANCY

If the egg had been fertilized, it would have implanted into the blood-thickened uterine lining which would sustain the embryo throughout the pregnancy.

Estrogen and progesterone are two of several hormones involved in a healthy pregnancy. Estrogen increases protein production to keep mother and child healthy. Along with progesterone and another hormone called **prolactin**, estrogen helps the mammary glands develop and causes nipple size to increase. Estrogen strengthens the uterine muscles which will be used during strong labor contractions. Also in preparation for labor, estrogen keeps the vaginal area soft and supple. In addition, estrogen alters its effect on collagen which then relaxes ligaments and joints, and causes body tissues to become soft and stretchy. This is essential for the actual child-bearing event, but such relaxing effects can cause problems in other parts of the body such as backaches or varicose veins.

Progesterone keeps the placenta functioning correctly for a healthy pregnancy. During the pregnancy, progesterone enters the baby's body and is converted into a group of hormones called the **corticosteroids** which control nutrient usage and how much salt and water is excreted in the urine. Progesterone helps prevent premature contractions and labor by decreasing the spasmodic motion of the uterine muscles. (This is called having an effect on the *smooth muscles* which are muscles over which we have no voluntary control. Smooth muscles are explained in more detail in Chapter 11.) In a negative way, this same smooth muscle effect can cause constipation and acid reflux. At the end of the pregnancy, progesterone levels fall, which brings on labor.

Throughout the pregnancy, these hormone levels may vary, affecting the mood centers in the brain, causing a full range of emotions including anger, depression, lethargy, and so many more.

HORMONES and MENOPAUSE

Because of erratic estrogen flows, a change in menstrual periods is usually the first indication of the onset of menopause. During perimenopause, periods will become irregular. (For a very small percentage of very fortunate women, this will be the only symptom that they are entering menopause.) As perimenopause progresses and finally culminates in the actual menopause, periods will be either heavy, light, and intermittent until, finally, no periods at all. Menopause is marked by the decrease in estrogen produced by the ovaries. However, they don't shut down all at once. Hormone production is sporadic for several years. Some months the ovaries will function normally, and other months they will not. After the ovarian estrogen stops, the adrenal glands will continue to secrete a hormone that is converted into estrogen in a woman's fat cells. This will continue, in varying amounts, for ten to twenty years.

In addition, as estrogen reduces and no longer overrides other sex hormones, menopause is marked by an increase in the **gonadotropin** hormones produced by the pituitary glands and higher amounts of the adrenally-produced **androgen** hormones (male hormones.)

A full discussion of hormones is the next chapter.

6
Women
Hormones In Your Body

HORMONES

So what exactly is a hormone? A hormone is a substance formed in some organ of the body and carried by a body fluid to another organ or tissue where it has a specific effect. The body uses various means to convey messages from one part to another. We are most familiar with nerve impulses ("electrical" messengers) and hormones, the chemical messengers. In fact, the actual word *hormone* comes from a Greek word meaning *to stimulate*. Both males and females have many hormones circulating throughout their body, and the following is a brief overview of some of these. Some of the terms are eye-popping, although most are simply descriptions of the hormone's function.

ESTROGEN

Estrogen is one of several female sex hormones produced primarily by the ovaries and, in smaller amounts, by a hormone secreted by the adrenal glands that is converted into estrogen in the fat tissues of the body. Ovarian-produced estrogen ceases at menopause. Adrenal production does not. Estrogen is what makes girls, girls. It causes females to have full breasts, soft skin, menstrual periods, and eggs that may be fertilized and become babies. Estrogen is necessary for strong bones and a healthy heart. But too much estrogen may raise the risk of breast or uterine cancer, contribute to the development of blood clots and gallstones, and exacerbate existing problems with fibrocystic breasts (chronically inflamed breast tissues) and uterine fibroids. When used as a part of Hormone Replacement Therapy, estrogen and progesterone together simulate a natural menstrual cycle.

Although we use the word *ESTROGEN* in a single sense, it is really a group of hormones. Specific estrogen hormones are estradiol, estrone and estriol. When the ovaries are still functioning at full force, before the menopause, they produce **estradiol**. This is converted into **estrone** and **estriol**. The estrogens contribute to a healthy female reproductive system. In the previous paragraph we learned that the adrenal glands secrete a hormone that is converted into estrogen in our fat cells. This is estrone, and it is the prevalent estrogen after the menopause. Estradiol and estrone are also produced synthetically and used in HRT.

PROGESTERONE

Progesterone is a female sex hormone secreted in the second half of the menstrual cycle by the corpus luteum in the ovaries. Progesterone gets its name from its essential role in the gestational process. A complete discussion of progesterone and the pregnancy process is in Chapter 5. Briefly, progesterone prepares and maintains the uterine lining to nurture a fertilized egg. It also helps develop the mammary glands, prevents premature labor, and helps initiate labor when it's time for the child to be born.

In addition to the corpus luteum within the ovary, progesterone is also produced in small amounts by the adrenal glands, and by the placenta during a pregnancy. (FYI: Small amounts of progesterone are produced in males in the testes.)

Without progesterone, women would have no menstrual periods. Increased production of progesterone after ovulation causes the uterine lining to thicken with blood cells in the event an egg is fertilized. If fertilization does not occur, production of both progesterone and estrogen decrease, and the uterine lining and the unfertilized egg are shed in the monthly period.

In hormone replacement therapy (HRT), progesterone combined with estrogen will simulate a natural menstrual cycle. Progesterone is also called **progestin**, which is a derivative of progesterone and is used synthetically in HRT. (see Chapter 18)

ANDROGEN HORMONES

Secreted by the adrenal glands, androgen hormones affect sex drive and growth in both men and women. They stimulate the development of characteristics we associate with the male sex such as facial and body hair, a deep voice and bulky muscles. In women, these hormones from the adrenal glands are less active and, therefore, do not usually cause a significant effect. However, as estrogen and progesterone from the ovaries begin to wane and no longer offset the androgens, unwelcome masculine traits may appear in women such as aggression, or an increase or darkening of facial hair.

TESTOSTERONE

Testosterone is the most active and important of the androgen hormones. It is what makes men, men. We are aware that testosterone is made in the testes of males. What isn't widely known is that small amounts of testosterone are also produced by the adrenal glands in both males and females, and by the ovaries in pre-menopausal women. These minute quantities in women contribute, in part, to sex drive and energy.

The production of testosterone and the other androgen hormones is controlled by the pituitary gland. An imbalance of testosterone in females can occasionally cause ovarian tumors or an increase in body hair.

GONADOTROPIN HORMONES

These are released by the pituitary gland and regulate the sex glands (gonads) in both men and women. Female gonads are ovaries and male gonads are the testes. Female and male fertility are controlled by the gonadotropins, which include the hormones FSH, LH, and HCG. (An explanation of these follow.)

LUTEINIZING HORMONE-RELEASING HORMONES (LH-RH)

Luteinizing hormone-releasing hormones are released by the hypothalamus when it senses low hormone levels. These chemicals are sent to the pituitary gland which then releases the gonadotropin hormones, FSH and LH. Gonadotropin hormones then regulate the production of the hormones *estrogen* and *androgen*. Organs stimulated by these sex hormones are the uterus, breasts and ovaries in women and the testes and prostate gland in men. The symptoms typically associated with menopause (hot flashes, irregular periods, etc.) may occur if there is a reduction or upset in these hormones.

FOLLICLE STIMULATING HORMONE (FSH)

The pituitary gland at the base of the brain produces the Follicle Stimulating Hormone (FSH) and the Luteinizing Hormone (LH). These are the most important of the gonadotropin hormones. FSH stimulates the development of eggs in the female and the development of testicular function in the male. FSH blood tests are used to detect levels of estrogen, progesterone and testosterone. If the FSH level is too high, there's usually a problem with the other hormones. FSH tests and estrogen levels are discussed at the conclusion of this chapter.

LUTEINIZING HORMONE (LH)

Along with the FSH, the Luteinizing Hormone (LH) is a gonadotropin hormone secreted by the pituitary gland. LH stimulates ovulation and, then, the development of the corpus luteum within the ovarian follicle so that it will secrete progesterone. The LH stimulates tissue development and testosterone secretions in the testes of men. (Lutein is associated with the color yellow, as found in vegetables.)

HORMONES PRESENT DURING PREGNANCY

The placenta produces hormones, including estrogen and progesterone, which help maintain that pregnancy. Some of these same hormones also affect menopausal women. We will look at them so you can see the connection.

1. Estrogen
2. Progesterone
3. **Prolactin** Secreted by the pituitary gland. Responsible for lactation functions including breast development and milk production during breastfeeding. Also stimulates some progesterone secretions. Name means *PRO* (*promoting*) + *LACT* (*lactation)*
4. **Human Placental Lactogen (HPL)** Secreted by the placenta. Responsible for lactation functions including breast enlargement and milk gland development. Breaks down fats in mother's body as energy source for developing fetus. Used to test for gestational diabetes because change in metabolism may result in imbalance in insulin levels.
5. **Melanocyte-stimulating Hormone (MSH)** Secreted by pituitary gland. In combination with estrogens, MSH stimulates skin pigmentation and

darkens nipples in pregnant women. May cause *chloasma* in both pregnant and menopausal women. (see Chapter 14)

6. **Human Chorionic Gonadotropin (HCG)** Secreted by the placenta. HCG is one of the gonadotropin hormones. HCG gets it name from the *chorion* which is the outer layer of cells that develops around the fertilized egg, from which the placenta develops. Acting similarly to the LH, HCG also stimulates the ovaries to produce estrogen and progesterone. HCG helps the mother's body adapt to pregnancy including preparing the breasts for lactation. Similar to HPL, HCG stimulates energy production for the fetus. Also similar to HPL, HCG may induce gestational diabetes. HCG production begins about ten days after conception and peaks at about 12 weeks. **Pregnancy tests** are based on detecting high levels of HCG in urine samples. Synthetic HCG, extracted from the urine of pregnant women, is used in the treatment of recurrent miscarriage and certain types of female and male infertility.

FSH Tests

The FSH is supposed to stimulate the follicle to ripen which makes the egg grow and releases a lot of estrogen. The estrogen is then supposed to tell the brain and pituitary to stop making FSH. But if the follicle doesn't ripen, no estrogen is produced, and no signal is received. So the FSH continues to be sent and sent and sent. A high FSH reading usually means a low level of estrogen. However, it's hard to determine accurate FSH levels for menopausal women because of the on again/off again estrogen flows. For women with permanently injured ovaries or women with Premature Ovarian Failure (POF), the FSH is a more reliable test. (POF is discussed in Chapter 10.)

Now, let's look at how menopause affects
the menstrual cycles..........

True Stories From Young Girls About Having Periods

After hearing the entire explanation of the menstrual cycle the young girl would soon be experiencing, she told her mother,
"No thanks. I'll pass."
(*Like it was an option!*)

Mother to ten-year old daughter: "So, honey, having periods will enable you to have babies when you grow up and get married."
Daughter to mother: "But since I'm not going to have any babies <u>now</u>, why fool with it?"
(*Out of the mouths of babes.*)

7

Menopause and Changes in Menstrual Cycles

MENSTRUAL CYCLE DESCRIPTIONS

Amenorrhea

Amenorrhea is the absence of menstrual periods due to disease, eating disorders, surgery, pregnancy, or menopause. There are two types of amenorrhea. *Primary amenorrhea* is due to an obvious cause such as pregnancy, menopause, disease, tumor or other medical disorder. *Secondary amenorrhea* may be due to excessive emotional stress or depression but is more usually caused by conditions that make the body to be in a starvation-like state such as the eating disorder anorexia nervosa, prolonged fasting or food deprivation, and/or excessive exercise. All these result in a hormonal imbalance and even a stoppage of the production of sex hormones. They also cause changes in metabolism, upsetting the body's chemistry. Whether the loss of periods is permanent or temporary depends on what brought on the amenorrhea in the first place. It will be temporary in the case of pregnancy or emotional stress while it is permanent in the case of hysterectomy and menopause.

CHANGES IN PERIODS DURING MENOPAUSE

A normal period is supposed to come along every 24-28 days. For some women, they are like clockwork. Of course, there are lots of women who have had irregular periods their entire life. In fact, it's "normal" for them to be irregular. Although it varies greatly from one woman to another, periods last around four days. Some women get a pinkish trickle or light discharge signal that they are about to start. Some women get no warning at all. The first day or two might be heavy followed by a general tapering off. However, once the pre-menopausal stage arrives, all this changes. Whether you were regular or regular in your irregularity, periods now will now run the full gamut of being either very heavy, very light, too often or too infrequent until, finally, your periods end completely.

NORMAL PERIOD ***(Menstruation)***

To have a normal period, there is a combination of normal estrogen flow + ovulation + normal progesterone flow which equals a normal endometrial lining.

HEAVY or LONG PERIOD ***(Menorrhagia)***
(excessive estrogen production)

Prolonged estrogen flow results in no ovulation. When there is no ovulation, no progesterone is produced. Without progesterone to curb it, the prolonged estrogen results in a very thick endometrial ling.

LIGHT or INFREQUENT PERIOD ***(Oligomenorrhea)***
(minimal estrogen production)

Too little estrogen results in no ovulation. No ovulation means no progesterone is produced. This low level of estrogen produces a thin endometrial lining.

NO PERIOD DUE TO MENOPAUSE ***(Amenorrhea)***
(no estrogen production)

No estrogen flow, no ovulation, no progesterone.

NO PERIOD DUE TO PREGNANCY*(Amenorrhea)*
During pregnancy, there is a normal estrogen flow + ovulation + fertilization + normal progesterone flow resulting in NO period.

PERIODS TOO OFTEN *(Polymenorrhea)*
When periods come more often than every 22 (or so) days.

PERIODS TOO EXTREME *(Metrorrhagia)*
Describes extremes in menstruation such as intervals between periods, length of time bleeding occurs, and the amount of blood expelled.

CONDITIONS RELATED TO CHANGES IN THE MENSTRUAL CYCLE

CRAMPS *(Dysmenorrhea)*
Painful cramps may be experienced during peri-menopause and menopause, even in women who never experienced cramping before. This pain and general discomfort is experienced during or just before the menstrual period. **Prostaglandins** are hormones secreted by the uterus which stimulate muscle spasms of the uterus and cause the blood-swollen uterine lining to shed in what we call menstruation. It is believed that an overproduction of prostaglandins causes excessive and prolonged contractions of the uterine muscles. The spasms can range from powerfully painful to a dull ache. These may be accompanied by headaches, migraines, lower-back aches, feeling bloated, nausea and even vomiting. Beside hormonal imbalances, cramping may be caused by endometriosis or fibroid tumors.

ENDOMETRIAL OVERGROWTH PROBLEMS
If there is no ovulation, no progesterone will be produced although estrogen will continue to be secreted. Without progesterone, there will no regular monthly cycle. Without this normal sloughing off of the uterine lining, the lining grows too thick due to uncontrolled estrogen flow, and can lead to problems such as:

ENDOMETRIAL HYPERPLASIA An enlargement of the uterine lining caused by an abnormal increase in the number of cells. This overgrowth of the uterine lining may be a forerunner of cancer.

ENDOMETRIAL CANCER A malignant tumor which often occurs due to too much estrogen which has caused an overgrown uterine lining. Usually requires surgery for partial or full removal of the uterus.

FIBROIDS A fibroid tumor is an abnormal growth that may occur inside or outside the walls of the uterus. Fibroids may grow as a result of prolonged estrogen flow. These tumors grow at variable rates but are almost always benign. Fibroids are usually found during routine pelvic examinations because, although most American women have them, few know it because there are often no symptoms, especially if the fibroid is small. (Fibroids range in size from as small as a pea to as large as a softball.) Symptoms of fibroid tumors include heavy menstrual bleeding, between-period spotting and/or anemia due to a heavy loss of blood during menses. One of the causes of fibroid tumors may be heredity. Also, a diet high in fats and red meats seems to stimulate the growth of fibroids. (Remember that estrogen conversion occurs primarily in the fat tissues.) Estrogen appears to make fibroids grow, especially during pregnancy when estrogen levels rise. After menopause, if the woman does not use hormone replacement therapy, fibroids usually shrink. Surgery to remove a fibroid only (but keep the uterus) is called a *myomectomy*. A *myoma* is a non-cancerous tumor of muscle.

CAUTION

Consult your doctor if you experience mid-cycle spotting. Although this can be common at the time of ovulation, it can also be a sign of endometriosis, uterine bleeding and/or fibroid tumors. For women who are over 40 years of age or who are menopausal, mid-cycle spotting can be a sign of polyps or uterine cancer.

If you started your periods when you were ten, and stop when you're 50, you would have had almost 500 periods.

Menopause is not a bad thing!

8
Statistics

Caution

You will notice that there aren't many statistics in the *Menopause Survival Guide*. Statistics are in a constant state of flux due to changes in population, available medical procedures, new drugs, etc. Many statistics are several years behind the current date because it takes a great deal of time and man-hours to compile data. The internet is the best source for current statistics. Go to a good search engine and type in the statistic you're interested in knowing. For example, if you want to know how many women have osteoporosis, just type in *osteoporosis statistics*. This will pull up a list of many sites. You may also be able to obtain information from your doctor.

There is a word of warning about statistics, though. Read them with a discerning eye. Statistics issued by a reputable organization such as the American Cancer Association, American Heart Association and the National Institute of Health are usually factual compilations of real data. These organizations have no hidden agenda, but this is not the case with all groups reporting statistics. Some statistics may be glossed over, over-rated or otherwise sensationalized in an effort to grab your attention and even separate you from your money. The media (papers, magazines, TV and radio) have found that scary statistics increase viewership. With more viewers, they are able to go to their sponsors and get more advertising revenue. The same may be true for manufacturers of certain products who may skew statistics to induce you to buy.

The best example of this is the media's distortion of the number of women at risk for breast cancer. Look at the following chart.
(Source: The National Cancer Institute.)

Age 25	1 in 19,608
Age 35	1 in 622
Age 45	1 in 93
Age 55	1 in 33
Age 65	1 in 17
Age 75	1 in 11
Age 85	1 in 9
Age 85 +	1 in 8

No reporter is going to read all these numbers. Long lists are boring and don't make good headlines. So they grab the one that's the most shocking. Guess which one? Yep, the 1 in 8 statistic. *One out of eight women are at risk for developing breast cancer over their lifetime.* Yikes! Sounds scary! But let's look at this a little more closely.

Did anyone explain that the phrase "lifetime risk" spans from birth to age 95? Covers a lot of ground, doesn't it? So, seriously, how many of us are going to make it to age 95? It just makes sense that if we live 95 years, we're probably going to get some kind of illness. And since at age 95, there aren't many people the same age around any more, the "risk per person" factor would certainly be working against us. But since all that wasn't explained, you've only gotten the tip of the statistical iceberg.

So get the entire iceberg. Do your homework and learn the full story. Don't go just by the headlines.

9

Estrogen and Cancer

Breast and Uterine Cancers

CANCER

The most common form of cancer is skin cancer. Of the non-skin cancers, the most common cancers in women are lung, breast, colon, and uterine (in that order.) But as frightening as cancer is, over the course of her lifetime, a woman has a much greater risk of developing heart disease, diabetes, alcoholism and then stroke before developing breast cancer. (Source: The National Cancer Institute)

Simply stated, cancer is when cells grow out of control. There are two types of tumors. One that isn't growing and won't spread is called **benign**. If it could spread throughout the body, it is called **malignant**. When the malignant cancer spreads from an initial area to another place in the body, it is called a **metastasis**. The location of the first tumor is called the *primary* cancer. The metastasis is a *secondary* malignant cancer. No matter where the primary cancer spreads, it will bear the name of that primary cancer. This means that if you have uterine cancer that spreads to the liver, the metastasis will be referred to as a uterine tumor in the liver. Cancer can spread through the body in the bloodstream, by spreading across tissues, and through the lymphatic system. (That's why lymph nodes are often removed, especially in breast cancer surgeries.)

Cancer can start for any reason: general wear and tear of life, chemicals, x-rays, environmental conditions, hormone imbalances, and who knows what all else. If we knew all the causes of all cancers, we would be able to do away with most of them. But even though we don't know all the causes, we do know some. For example, everyone is aware of the connection between cigarette smoking and lung cancer. Of particular interest to readers of the *Menopause Survival Guide* is the link between breast and uterine cancers and menopause.

BREAST CANCER

BREAST CANCER. Two of the world's scariest words. This disease is often associated with menopausal women, especially those who have taken hormone replacement therapy (HRT), but it can strike anyone at any time. (Men can get breast cancer, too.) Even without HRT, you are considered at high-risk for breast cancer if you have an immediate relative who has had breast cancer, if you smoke, are overweight, started your period before age 12, had children after age 30, or never bore children. Some women have a history of breast or ovarian cancer in their family and may have specific gene mutations that put them at a higher lifetime risk for both breast and ovarian cancer. (If you see the term *first-degree relative*, that means a sister, mother, daughter, grandmother, or aunt.)

BREASTS

Although they come in a variety of sizes and shapes, all breasts are composed of the same stuff. There are about 15-20 *milk glands* (or *lobules*) with tube-like structures called *ducts* which transport the milk. The rest of the breast is composed of *fatty tissue*. Providing structure for the breast and giving it shape are thin *ligaments* that are interwoven between the glands and the fat cells. Although the breast is connected to the pectoral (chest) muscle, the breast itself contains no muscle. It is, in fact, mainly fat.

DENSE BREASTS

If you have a higher proportion of milk glands and ducts than fat tissue, your breasts are "dense." High breast density is often on the *increased risk for breast cancer* list. You cannot see or feel the density yourself, but it is readily evident on mammograms. (Density has nothing to do with the size or shape of a breast.)

The number of glands in relation to fat tissue is important because most breast cancers develop in or on the milk glands and ducts. The more glands and ducts, the more places for problems to pop up. So you would think that having fewer glands might work in your favor in avoiding breast cancer. However, there is another catch.

THE FAT FACTOR

We know that the ovaries have been pumping out estrogen since we were in the womb. In addition, from puberty through menopause, the adrenal glands have also been producing a hormone that is converted into estrogen in our fat cells. At menopause, there is an increased amount of this estrogen conversion which may continue, in varying amounts, for 10-20 years after menopause. Knowing that estrogen conversion occurs primarily in fat tissues, and knowing that the breast is primarily fat, is another explanation for why breast cancer is so prevalent. The breast is like an estrogen magnet.

Fat affects estrogen levels in both younger AND older women because fat cells step up estrogen production. After menopause, when ovaries stop making estrogen, fat becomes a major factor in how much estrogen circulates in a woman's blood. A higher level of estrogen equals an increased risk of breast cancer. This explains why studies have found that being overweight and being physically inactive can raise your risk for breast cancer, even if you have never taken one estrogen supplement in your life. That's not to say that skinny women who never exercise don't get breast cancer, because they do. But overweight and/or inactive women face a greater risk.

BREAST CANCER and EXERCISE

The fat factor is obvious. The more body fat, the more places estrogen can come to roost. But why physical activity? It is proven that physical activity accelerates all movement throughout our system; e.g., food flows through our digestive system faster when we are physically active. Exercise has also proven to affect the circulating estrogen in a woman's body which means it doesn't stay as long in one part of the body. It is believed that exercise decreases the breast tissue's amount of exposure to circulating estrogen, which may lower the risk of breast cancer.

SYMPTOMS and PREVENTIVE MEASURES

So maintaining a healthy weight and being physically active probably will lower your risk of getting breast cancer. Other tried and true preventive measures still hold. Do a monthly breast self-examination. Most lumps are first found by the woman herself, not a doctor or x-ray. Be aware of any changes in the look and feel of your breast. Lumps, discoloration, dimpling, even unusual itching are symptoms that should be investigated. Have a yearly pap smear at which time your doctor will check for breast lumps or other suspicious symptoms. Imaging procedures like body scans and mammograms are excellent diagnostic tools for detecting breast abnormalities. And before you panic too much should you find a lump, be aware that most lumps aren't cancerous. But do have anything unusual checked out. Remember that early detection saves lives.

LUMPS

If you do find a lump, don't automatically think that you've got cancer. Breasts are lumpy by nature. During menstrual cycles, they get lumpier due to hormonal changes. And during menopause, they also get lumpier from natural estrogen fluctuations or estrogen replacement therapy. Most non-cancerous lumps (cysts) are smooth, firm, and easily moved with the fingertips. Cancerous lumps are usually hard and aren't easily moved. HOWEVER, have your doctor check out each and every lump. Don't take any chances.

BE PERSISTENT

If you think something is amiss in your breast, be persistent. If your doctor dismisses your fears even though you KNOW something is wrong, INSIST you are thoroughly checked. Get a second opinion, if necessary. *One woman had a weird symptom: Whenever she took a shower, she got a shiny, white spot on her breast, and it itched. The spot would disappear after her skin dried and cooled. But it happened each time she showered. Her family doctor dismissed the symptoms because her most recent mammogram had indicated no bad spots. She waited a while, but when it didn't go away, she insisted on another mammogram. Guess what. There WAS a spot.* She knew her own breast. She knew something had changed. Her doctor didn't listen. Surgery took care of the lump because this woman was smart enough to take care of her own health!

HRT and BREAST CANCER

Now, concerning HRT and breast cancer. Nearly every study has shown that HRT does increase the risk of breast cancer. Some women have opted to take that chance in favor of what they consider to be the benefits of HRT. These pros and cons are all discussed in Chapter 18. You must learn all you can about HRT and breast cancer, and then decide for yourself what is right for you. Listen to the suggestions and advice of doctors, friends, and your family. Then decide for yourself. It's your breast. It's your life. It's your decision.

BREAST SURGERIES

A mastectomy is a general term referring to the removal of a breast. The old method of treating any breast cancer was to lop off the entire breast, remove all the chest muscles from collar bone to belly button, and scoop out most of the underarm area where the lymph nodes are. In nearly every case, it was surgical "overkill", and the woman was left with a ravaged body. However, with new procedures and with new consideration for the woman involved, these radical mastectomies are rarely performed. The goal now is to remove all the cancerous areas in a way that is the least invasive. Here are descriptions of the various surgeries:

Mastectomy Generic term for the removal of the entire breast.
Simple mastectomy Removal of the entire breast and some of the underarm lymph nodes.
Radical mastectomy Removal of the entire breast, chest muscles, and all underarm (axillary) lymph nodes.
Quadrantectomy 1/4 of the breast is removed.
Lumpectomy Removal of breast lump only.
Axillary sampling Removal of some of the underarm lymph nodes.
Radical axillary clearance Removal of all the underarm lymph nodes.

Although the initial diagnosis can be scary as can be, statistics indicate that breast cancer is not necessarily a death sentence. Especially with early detection, the long-term survival rate is quite good. (Talk to your doctor about exact statistics.) As with all cancers, there are many treatment options such as surgery, chemotherapy, radiation, medication, and others. The oncologist (cancer doctor) will be able to explain all your options, and then you can decide which treatment, if any, is best for you.

UTERINE CANCER (specifically, ENDOMETRIAL CANCER)

Just like the breast, the lining of the uterus (the endometrium) is an estrogen magnet. When a woman has a normal menstrual cycle, estrogen makes the uterine lining swell with blood. Halfway through the cycle, if there is no pregnancy, progesterone curbs the flow of estrogen, and the uterine lining sheds. When hormonal fluctuations begin in preparation for menopause, this process is disrupted. Without ovulation, there is no progesterone to counterbalance, and then stem, the estrogen production. So estrogen continues to flow, uncontrolled by progesterone, and the result is a very thick endometrial lining. When this thick uterine lining is not sloughed off as it would be during a menstrual cycle, it is soon overgrown. This can lead to problems like **fibroids** and **endometrial hyperplasia**. Sadly, it may also result in endometrial cancer. Most uterine cancers are in the uterine lining. (Some cancers are also in the cervix.) In most cases, when uterine cancer is diagnosed, the uterus is removed in an operation called a **hysterectomy**. Hysterectomies are discussed in more detail in Chapter 10. As with breast cancer, early detection and treatment means that a diagnosis of uterine cancer is not an automatic death sentence.

Because of the uncontrolled estrogen flow associated with menopause, uterine cancer occurs most often in women over age 50. In addition, a post-menopausal woman who is 50 or more pounds overweight has an even higher risk of developing uterine cancer because of the connection between body fat and estrogen production. As discussed earlier in this chapter, the adrenal glands produce a hormone that is converted into estrogen in fat cells. Obese women have a higher level of circulating estrogen than women who are not overweight. This excess estrogen comes to roost in the endometrial lining (and the breast.) Also at risk for uterine cancer are women who have had few or no children. (This is because every time a woman gives birth, it's like a big house-cleaning in the uterine area.)

SYMPTOMS

Symptoms of uterine cancer can include heavy vaginal bleeding in menstrual women, and a bleeding, vaginal discharge in menopausal women. Unlike cervical cancer, uterine cancer is not detected in a pap smear. (Neither is ovarian cancer.) As a means of prevention, progesterone is often given to offset the estrogen flow.

HRT and ENDOMETRIAL CANCER

When estrogen replacement is taken, it is usually accompanied by progesterone to offset the estrogen flow and subsequent buildup of the uterine lining.

CAUTION

If you suspect there might be anything at all wrong symptom-wise, it is important to see your doctor right away as early detection is the key to long-term survival of victims of uterine cancer. If it's caught early enough, the cancerous uterus may be removed before cancer cells spread to other parts of the body.

10
Estrogen and Non-Natural Menopause

Surgery Chemotherapy Radiation
Premature Ovarian Failure

A woman usually enters the menopausal stage as a natural part of the aging process. However, menopause can be brought on by surgery, medications, or treatments such as chemotherapy. Frequently this happens years and even decades before she should naturally enter menopause. This is called **non-natural**, **surgical** or **induced menopause**.

We'll discuss some of these.

SURGICAL MENOPAUSE:
Hysterectomy and Oophorectomy

The two operations most associated with menopause are hysterectomy and oophorectomy. **Hysterectomy** is the removal of the uterus. **Oophorectomy** is the removal of one or both of the ovaries. *A unilateral oophorectomy* refers to the removal of just one ovary. A *bilateral oophorectomy* refers to the removal of both ovaries. Hysterectomy and oophorectomy are distinct operations. Having one does not mean the other is automatically performed. However, it is often standard operating procedure for the ovaries to be removed when the uterus is removed. We'll talk more about this later.

Periods will stop when either organ is removed. No uterus NO PERIOD because there would be no place for the menstrual cycle to "grow." No ovaries NO PERIOD because you need at least one ovary to release an egg to stimulate that "growth" of the menstrual cycle in the uterus.

Having or not having a uterus has NOTHING to do with estrogen production. Having or not having an ovary has EVERYTHING to do with estrogen production. And it is the waning and eventual shutting down of ovarian estrogen production that determines natural menopause. Surgical removal of the uterus and the subsequent cessation of periods is a case of **amenorrhea** (no periods) rather than age-related menopause that causes periods to cease.

If the uterus only is removed at an age before the woman would naturally enter menopause, she will not experience the classic menopausal symptoms because her ovaries are still producing normal amounts of estrogen. But with or without her uterus, when she reaches her 40's to 50's, menopausal symptoms will start as her ovaries begin to produce less and less estrogen. But no matter her age, if a woman has surgery to remove the uterus AND both ovaries, she will be thrown into instant menopause and experience all the symptoms associated with it.

OOPHORECTOMY

Throughout our life, our ovaries manufacture estrogen, progesterone, and small amounts of testosterone (which heightens sexual desire.) Even after menopause, the ovaries continue to secrete very small amounts of these for a while. But in surgical menopause due to an oophorectomy, all these hormones stop "cold turkey". The small amount of estrogen stimulated by the adrenal glands just isn't enough to make much difference. Since there is not enough estrogen to counterbalance other hormones, higher amounts of the gonadotropin hormones (produced by pituitary gland) and of the androgens (male hormones) will be present in the bloodstream. This can result in problems such as facial hair growth discussed in Chapter 14.

HYSTERECTOMY

Hysterectomy is the second most common operation on women (Cesarean sections are first.) By age 60, one in three women will have had their uterus removed. This is not always a good thing. No surgery should be entered into lightly, and this is no exception. However, many women consider a hysterectomy the best thing they ever did. For women who suffer with incredibly heavy bleeding and the painful spasms associated with it, they look upon a hysterectomy as a blessing. Of course, in the case of cancer or pre-cancerous conditions, the removal of the uterus is usually a necessity. There should always be careful thought concerning whether or not the ovaries will be removed at the time of the removal of the uterus.

AT HIGHER RISK

Women who have these surgeries may be put at a higher risk for problems than women going through natural menopause. Most of these are associated with the premature loss of ovarian-produced estrogen. This is a double-edged sword because the woman's body has not had as much time to experience the benefits associated with natural estrogen production, AND she suffers longer with the effects of estrogen depletion. After having both a bilateral oophorectomy and a hysterectomy, women may experience higher levels of bad cholesterol and high blood pressure than if they had had a hysterectomy alone and kept their ovaries.

Also, women who had a hysterectomy before the natural age for menopause may be at a higher risk for coronary heart disease for the rest of her life. In addition to estrogen loss, when the uterus is removed, a woman loses the benefits of **prostaglandins.** These are fatty acids secreted by the uterus, and they control the stickiness of blood platelets. Without these, blood clots form more easily, increasing a risk of blockages in the bloodstream which heightens the risk of heart disease and stroke. Other side effects associated with hysterectomy or oophorectomy may include chronic pain associated with internal scar tissue. Depression may also be a serious psychological effect because of the actual physical loss of the female organs, and the loss of fertility and womanhood associated with them.

CHEMOTHERAPY, RADIATION and MEDICATION

Women may also be thrown into early menopause when the ovaries are damaged or destroyed as a result of chemotherapy or radiation therapy, and even some medications. The effects and risks are the same as those discussed for oophorectomies.

PREMATURE OVARIAN FAILURE (POF)

Premature Ovarian Failure is a disorder that may be mistakenly diagnosed as early menopause. Although the symptoms may be the same, the causes are quite different. First a little female biology. Within the ovaries are three to four hundred thousand follicles. These are microscopic sacs that contain undeveloped eggs. During a normal menstrual cycle, the Follicle Stimulating Hormone (FSH) will stimulate the follicle to grow and to produce estrogen. When it is mature, the follicle will burst and the egg will shoot out. During menopause, the ovaries eventually run out of developable follicles meaning eggs no longer grow and estrogen is no longer being released.

However, in the case of POF, the ovaries still have these primitive follicles, but they just don't function correctly. This is called *follicle dysfunction.*

What causes POF is unknown. In most cases, it simply comes on spontaneously. In a small number of cases, there may be some link with heredity or an autoimmune disorder. Some women may begin to experience POF after surgery, radiation or chemotherapy. Some women were simply born with a shortage of follicles. What is known is that POF brings on menopausal symptoms in women far too young to be experiencing actual menopause. Since this disorder is relatively unknown, it is often misdiagnosed, although many women are believed to have it.

Testing levels of FSH (the follicle stimulating hormone) may help diagnose POF but you cannot get an instant diagnosis as levels have to be tested several times. Estrogen levels may be high at first, but later diminish. The FSH is used to test for levels of estrogen, progesterone and testosterone. High levels of FSH are reached this way. The FSH is supposed to stimulate the follicle to ripen, which makes the egg grow and to release a lot of estrogen. The estrogen is then supposed to tell the brain and pituitary to stop making FSH. But if the follicle doesn't ripen, no estrogen is produced, and no signal is received. So the FSH continues to be sent and sent and sent. It's hard to determine accurate FSH levels for menopausal women because of the on again/off again estrogen flows. For women with permanently injured ovaries or women with Premature Ovarian Failure, the FSH is a more reliable test. POF is defined when a woman has had no period for four months and when at least two FSH tests have been taken, at least one month apart, with FSH levels between 30 and 40 (depending on your doctor.)

A woman experiencing Premature Ovarian Failure will have menstrual periods that either cease or become intermittent, and hot flashes, night sweats and other symptoms similar to menopause. Although most women with POF are unable to conceive, it is not an impossibility. Because ovarian function may be intermittent, pregnancy could unexpectedly occur, even many years after the first diagnosis. Treatment is usually for the woman to take some form of HRT until she reaches the age when menopause would normally occur. However, as with all HRT treatment, women should be advised to learn all the risks and benefits associated with HRT.

There are excellent informational sites and support groups on the internet. Do a search for *POF* or *Premature Ovarian Failure.*

HRT & NON-NATURAL MENOPAUSE

Hormone Replacement Therapy is usually taken up until a time when natural menopause would have occurred. This is not a requirement, of course, and carries all the benefits and risks of HRT that are discussed in Chapter 18. When the uterus only is removed, HRT is not usually necessary because the ovaries are still producing estrogen. If both ovaries are removed, HRT will be offered. If only one ovary is removed, HRT may not be necessary.

11
Estrogen and Elasticity / Muscle Strength

Gravity and estrogen depletion can create serious problems concerning the elasticity of tissues and muscle strength. This happens on both the outside AND inside of our body.

ELASTICITY and MUSCLE STRENGTH

You know what happens when the elastic on a pair of socks loses its stretchiness and gets worn out. It looks misshapen, and it won't hold our socks up any more. They droop or fall down around our ankles. The same sagging and wrinkling occurs when reduced estrogen levels in our body decrease the elasticity in the skin's connective tissue. It can also produce a loss of muscle strength, which in turn can have deteriorating effects on certain organs. These effects have always been associated with aging but, of course, we lose estrogen as we age, so they are all tied in to-gether. Let's look first at the different types of muscles in our body, and then at conditions that we may experience as muscles change due to estrogen loss.

MUSCLES (*Three types*)

There are three types of muscles. **Skeletal muscles** are those under the *voluntary* control of the brain. That means we can consciously control their movement. For example, flexing our arm muscles, making a fist, smiling, or pointing a finger. **Cardiac muscle** is found only in the heart. **Smooth muscles** are also called *involuntary* muscles. Their nerve supply comes from the autonomic nervous system, and they are not under our conscious control. (The *autonomic nervous system* is the part of our body that automatically runs on its own, without us having to tell it what to do. It controls functions like heart pumping and lung breathing.) All muscles respond to changes in hormones, oxygen levels, nutrients, etc.

In addition to muscles, our ligaments and connective tissues (such as tendons and cartilage) all have an elastic quality. They can contract and expand to some degree. But over time, decreased estrogen levels can lead to a loss of this elasticity. Outwardly, we can see when shoulders begin to droop, and when wrinkles and jowls start to appear. However, this same process is happening to parts we can't see. That's why we may develop such undesirable conditions as Bladder Incontinence, Uterine Prolapse, and Vaginal Atrophy, which are as unpleasant as their names imply. These conditions usually begin during the perimenopause stage and may get progressively worse as we age.

BLADDER INCONTINENCE

Urinary incontinence is when you urinate when you don't want to. This uncontrolled, totally involuntary urination may be due to injury, disease or, in the case of menopausal women, caused by hormonal changes. When low estrogen levels affect the smooth muscle of the tissues lining the urethra, they become thin and stretched, which reduces bladder support. There are several types of incontinence, but the one most applicable to Change of Lifers is *stress incontinence,* which is the involuntary escape of small amounts of urine when a woman sneezes, laughs, coughs, picks up something heavy or participates in strenuous physical activities. This incontinence is caused when the sphincter muscles around the urethra weaken and lose their "elastic" quality. (A *sphincter* is a ring of muscle around an opening that opens and closes like a valve to regulate inflow/outflow.) Besides accidental leakage, you may also feel frequently like you need to empty your bladder. As if all this wasn't embarrassing and annoying enough, a sagging bladder is also much more prone to infections such as cystitis. Because incontinence is usually due to hormonal changes, women will be affected more than men, and the elderly more than younger women. Stress incontinence is also common in women who have just undergone vaginal childbirth because the same sphincter muscles become stretched during childbirth.

Urge incontinence sudden urge to urinate
Stress incontinence involuntary leakage
Overflow incontinence constant leaking of small amounts of urine

So, short of surgery, what can you do? Keep the bladder empty as much as is possible to prevent accidental leakage. Kegel exercises may help regain strength in the muscles associated with bladder incontinence. Kegel's are explained later in this chapter.

EXCEPTION TO THE RULE.......

Our ability to consciously control holding urination or a bowel movement is one of the few exceptions to the voluntary/involuntary muscle story. We are able to have SOME say in when we "go" or need to "hold" going to the bathroom although, as we all know, the actions ARE going to happen eventually.

CONSTIPATION

Constipation may also develop due to the loss of rectal muscle tone. Gas and constipation may occur as the entire gastro-intestinal tract slows down due to changes in metabolism.

DRY SKIN, WRINKLES and ACNE

Estrogen loss is one of the main culprits responsible for wrinkles and dry skin. Estrogen and progesterone stimulate the sebaceous glands in the skin to produce sebum. *Sebum* is an oily secretion composed of fats and waxes which keeps skin soft and supple, prevents us from becoming soggy when wet, protects our skin from cracking when exposed to dry conditions, and puts up a defensive barrier against outside "bad guys" like bacteria and harmful forms of fungus. When estrogen and progesterone decrease, the skin's natural oils diminish causing the skin to become dry and thin. Most studies indicate that women who use estrogen replacement have fewer wrinkles and are less likely to have dry skin. By the same token, these hormone fluctuations during menopause can cause excessively oily skin, and even *acne.* if the sebaceous glands are overstimulated. This acne usually diminishes as the hormone production subsides.

HAIR THINNING or LOSS

Estrogen loss can cause slower sebum production in the scalp, diminishing natural oils, and making the skin on the head become thinner and less elastic. This slows down the growth of hair, making it weak and of poor quality. As the scalp hair (and other body hair) becomes dry and brittle, it may come out easily. Although hair loss or thinning hair is usually considered an issue for men, this is a real concern for many women, especially those of menopausal age.

INDIGESTION, HEARTBURN and ACID REFLUX

Changes in the gastro-intestinal tract and loss of muscle strength in the esophagus can contribute to indigestion and heartburn brought on by acid reflux, which happens when acid from the stomach flows back into the esophagus.

STRETCH MARKS

Stretch marks, medically known as *stria,* are caused by a lack of elasticity and thinning in the skin. Stria may be caused by a hormone imbalance that affects collagen in the skin. They appear on the hips and thighs of teenage girls, and are most often associated with pregnant women who get them on their breasts, thighs, and on their lower torso where the skin has stretched to accommodate the growing baby. If a woman isn't already loaded up with them by the time she hits menopause, stretch marks will probably only be a concern if she gains or loses a great deal of weight because her skin won't be able to adapt to her body's changing shape as readily as if she still had the elasticity provided by sufficient estrogen.

UTERINE PROLAPSE *(descensus)*

There are ligaments that support the uterus and hold it in place. When these ligaments get stretched during childbirth, or lose their strength due to estrogen loss during menopause, the uterus may begin to descend from its normal position. This may be minor at first, but could eventually result in the uterus actually protruding through the vaginal opening. In the early stages, there may be no symptoms other than a general feeling that something just doesn't feel right "down there." If the disorder is allowed to progress too long, the uterus may actually push out when the woman strains during physical activity or a hard bowel movement. (Except in an advanced stage, the uterus will retract back into the body.) Surgery is usually required to repair this condition. The same Kegel exercises that helped with incontinence can also help prevent or, at least, deter uterine prolapse. The word *descensus* refers to the *descending* of the uterus.

VAGINAL ATROPHY and DRYNESS

For many menopausal women, vaginal dryness is a major complaint. Once again, this is due to estrogen loss. Before menopause, estrogen kept the vaginal walls thick, elastic, and moist. When estrogen levels fall, secretions diminish and the vaginal skin thins. Over time, the vagina shrinks (atrophy), becoming shorter, narrower, and drier resulting in painful and difficult sex. These changes also make the vagina more prone to minor infections. For the dryness, there are over-the-counter remedies available that provide unobtrusive, simple lubrication. Hormone replacement therapy and even some herbal remedies will usually diminish this frustrating side effect of menopause.

VAGINAL PROLAPSE

The estrogen effect can cause vaginal prolapse which occurs when either the front or back vaginal wall moves from its proper placement. Like vaginal atrophy, this condition can also cause painful sex. Vaginal prolapse can be corrected surgically by either a *cystocele*, *rectocele* or *urethrocele*. (see Glossary)

KEGEL (perineal) EXERCISES

Perineal exercises are best known as *Kegel exercises.* To do these, pretend that you have to urinate but you're not near a bathroom. Tighten the same muscles you would if you had to "hold" it for a while. (These are the perineal muscles.) Several series of these tightenings are the basis of the Kegel exercises. Doing them daily is a good preventive measure for women of all ages. After any damage has occurred because of estrogen loss, Kegel's may help regain strength in the perineal muscles.

Here's a Thought About Aging

God probably designed it so that our eyesight
fails as we get older,
especially so that we can't see
very good up close.
That way, we can't see wrinkles or
age spots on our mate.
In our mind's eye,
they look just as young as when
we married them.

12
Estrogen and Heart Disease Estrogen and Stroke

HEART DISEASE and STROKE

The flow of blood is what keeps us alive. When the flow to the heart is impaired, we call it a **heart attack**. When the flow to the brain is impaired, we call it a **stroke.** The major cause of both of these conditions is **atherosclerosis**. Let's take a quick overview of these familiar terms. Then we'll look at how they are linked to estrogen, estrogen loss, and estrogen replacement.

The leading causes of death in women are heart disease, cancer, and stroke.

HEART ATTACK

Heart attacks are just one of many types of heart disorders or heart diseases, and impaired blood supply is the major cause of most heart problems. The medical community has a long list of specific terms and conditions relating to heart problems, but the general public just calls it a heart attack when the heart stops working. Let's look at the medical side of things. The heart is a muscle that rhythmically pumps blood to the rest of our body. When this rhythmic, muscular activity stops for any number of reasons, and the pumping of blood suddenly stops, this is called **cardiac arrest.** Heart attack, medically called **myocardial infarction,** is the most common cause of cardiac arrest. A heart attack is when a part of the heart muscle suddenly dies due to an interruption in its blood supply. Because of a blockage in an artery or vein in the heart, that part of the heart suddenly dies (heart attack.) That causes the rest of the heart muscle to stop pumping blood (cardiac arrest.) Impaired blood supply may be due to a number of conditions including infections, tumors, injuries, a damaged heart valve, and congenital defects, but the most common cause is *atherosclerosis*.

The classic symptoms of heart attack are cold, clammy skin, restlessness, nausea, vomiting, shortness of breath, or loss of consciousness. Other symptoms may include weakness or unexplained fatigue, or a feeling of impending doom. In most cases, the actual attack is accompanied by a crushing, continuous chest pain that may radiate into the back, left arm, and left jaw. Symptoms leading up to a heart attack may be mild to severe, although sometimes there will be no pain at all and only when tests are run at a later date will it be revealed that the person suffered a heart attack.

STROKE

Stroke is damage to the brain caused by blood leaking outside the vessel walls or by an interruption to the brain's blood supply. Strokes are fatal in about 1/3 of the cases, cause permanent dysfunction in 1/3 of the cases, and result in no long-lasting ill effects in 1/3 of the cases. Whether there is a loss in feeling, movement, speech, or bodily function will be dependent on what part of the brain was injured and to what extent. Hypertension, atherosclerosis, and sudden blockages in the bloodstream are the primary causes leading to stroke. **Hypertension** (high blood pressure) weakens the arterial walls. **Atherosclerosis** is a thickening and narrowing of the lining of the walls of the arteries. (see discussion in next paragraph.) Blockages occur when a small particle called an

embolus travels through the bloodstream, becomes lodged in a vessel, and blocks blood flow. These particles can be blood clots, bubbles of air or gas, pieces of tissue or tumor, bacteria, bone marrow, fat or cholesterol. When an embolus causes a blockage, it is called an **embolism**. The buildup of plaque in atherosclerosis may "grab" one of these emboli, or it may be a piece of plaque itself that breaks off and becomes the embolus.

Symptoms of stroke include slurred speech, loss of speech, headache, dizziness, confusion, double vision or temporary blindness, difficulty swallowing, and/or weakness or paralysis on one side of the body. A **Transient Ischemic Attack (TIA)** is a stroke in which symptoms last fewer than 24 hours and which is followed by a full recovery. TIA's are a warning sign of a problem and must be investigated. Stroke is the leading cause of serious, long-term disability in the United States.

ATHEROSCLEROSIS

The most common cause of both heart attack and stroke is atherosclerosis. This is very much like the buildup in a drain pipe. As soap residue, minerals, hairs, and other stuff flows through a drain pipe, some of it sticks to the walls of the pipes. But it doesn't stick in a smooth, slick layer. Instead it sticks in little peaks and valleys. The peaks act as hooks that "grab" more fats, hairs, and other bad stuff as they are drained from the sink and, eventually, you have a clogged drain. Atherosclerosis works the same way. The inner layer of the arterial wall thickens due to the formation of raised places called **plaque**. This reduces the size of the artery and impairs blood flow. Plaques are little spots of fats, decaying cells, clumps of blood platelets, cholesterol, or calcium. As the smooth lining of the blood vessel thickens, blood clots may be formed which can break off, travel through the blood stream, and block smaller veins and arteries. When the coronary arteries, which supply blood to the heart, become narrowed due to atherosclerosis and parts of the heart muscle are deprived of oxygen, a **heart attack** can occur. When any arteries to the brain are blocked, a **stroke** can occur.

THE ESTROGEN CONNECTION

So, how is all of this related to menopause and the decrease in estrogen? Up to age 60, men die of heart attacks at six times the rate of women. By age 70, that ratio equals. Most of this is because of estrogen loss. Even though estrogen production falls while women are in their 40's and 50's, some of the effects of the decrease in this hormone may not show up for years. Others, of course, can be noticed much sooner. Some of the risks associated with heart disease and stroke are high blood pressure, high levels of bad cholesterol, blood clots, and weak veins and heart muscles. All of these are affected by the loss of estrogen in some way.

Estrogen directly affects our internal body chemistry, what we call **metabolism**. This causes a rise in blood pressure, and an increase in fats in the blood. Both can lead to an increase in atherosclerosis (fatty deposits in arteries) and an increased chance of coronary heart disease and stroke. The connection between fat and estrogen is discussed in more detail in Chapter 9.

Estrogen can also affect the heart directly. The heart is a muscle, and all muscles respond to changes in hormones, oxygen levels, nutrients, etc. Just like all of the other parts in our body, the heart is affected by the loss of **elasticity** in muscles, connective tissues, and ligaments, brought about by estrogen decreases. (see Chapter 11)

Estrogen helps keep **calcium** in the bones. Calcium is also important in maintaining the smooth muscle of the heart (the cardiac muscle) because it affects the tension in the heart walls which in turn affects the pumping ability of the heart.

As estrogen falls with menopause, many women gain weight and their blood pressure rises. Many post-menopausal women have higher levels of triglycerides, overall **cholesterol** and LDL (bad) cholesterol because of the decrease in estrogen which once helped keep cholesterol levels balanced. HRT appears to raise levels of HDL (good cholesterol) and lower the LDL.

Risk for stroke and heart attack also increases after menopause, and especially after a hysterectomy. The uterus secretes **prostaglandins** which are fatty acids that act like hormones. One of the effects of certain prostaglandins is that they reduce the stickiness of blood platelets. With the removal of the uterus, this production of prostaglandins decreases, and blood clots form more easily, increasing the risk of stroke and heart attack.

REAL SYMPTOMS or MIMICS?

If the possibility of these real illnesses isn't enough, estrogen fluctuations and the anxiety associated with menopause can mimic most of the symptoms of heart attack or stroke. Irregular amounts of estrogen acting upon the autonomic nervous system can quicken the heart beat and breathing rate. A low level of estrogen may trigger the nerves in the heart muscle when tense or tired which can cause a pounding or **palpitating** sensation. In addition, emotional tension can cause muscle spasms, even in the heart muscle. **Shortness of breath**, chest pains, and numbness or tingling in the extremities are frequent complaints of menopausal women. Since these are also symptoms of heart attack and stroke, they are nothing to ignore. Do not hesitate to have any symptom checked out thoroughly to rule out any threatening medical condition. But should a full battery of tests turn up nothing wrong, there is every possibility that estrogen fluctuations and/or stress may be causing your symptoms!

HYPERVENTILATION

Hyperventilation is panting, or abnormally deep, rapid breathing. Although it may be caused by any number of medical conditions, it is usually a result of anxiety or strenuous exercise. Hyperventilation is brought on by an imbalance in the amount of oxygen and carbon dioxide in the bloodstream. One of the things that controls our rate of breathing is the level of carbon dioxide in the bloodstream. When our body is overworked physically, or when we are under too much stress, the amount of carbon dioxide increases quickly in the bloodstream which causes us to breathe more rapidly in an effort to eliminate that carbon dioxide and take in more oxygen.

Because of the oxygen deficiency in the bloodstream, symptoms of hyperventilation include faintness and the feeling of an inability to take a full breath. In your hands and feet you may feel numbness, tingling, or even spasms or twitches. **Tetany** is the name for this annoying and sometimes painful twitching that is often common in the facial areas of the eye, upper lip, and cheek in times of stress. Since these symptoms are also the same as those for heart attack or stroke, all these effects can add to the already existing feeling of anxiety. Sufferers often experience a feeling of impending doom which is another symptom shared with heart attacks. Other aggravating but harmless effects of hyperventilation are **sighing** and **yawning**. Although usually associated with being sleepy or bored, these may actually be caused by high levels of carbon dioxide in the blood, and sighing and yawning are efforts by the body to reduce the carbon dioxide level in the bloodstream and increase the oxygen level.

ANGINA

Angina may also be brought on by the menopausal effect. Shortened from the medical term **Angina Pectoris**, Angina is chest pain caused by a lack of oxygen to the heart muscle, frequently a result of poor blood supply. Pain usually comes on when the heart is working harder and requires more oxygen; e.g., when exercising or under stress. Symptoms include a sensation of pressure in the chest, throat, upper jaw, back, between the shoulder blades or in the arms. Other symptoms may include nausea, sweating, dizziness, and breathing difficulty. Once again, since these are the same symptoms as heart attack or stroke, consult your doctor.

HRT, HEART DISEASE and STROKE

There is certainly considerable debate whether estrogen replacement therapy during menopause lessens or actually increases the risk of heart disease. Where it may help with calcium and the smooth muscle effect, it may increase the risk of cardiovascular disease in women with atherosclerosis. HRT also does not appear to reduce the risk of stroke in women who have previously had strokes or TIA's. Please talk to your physician for complete information.

The best way to avoid heart attack and stroke is to follow sensible guidelines such as maintaining a healthy weight, exercising, not smoking, and keeping stress to a minimum. Learn more by contacting your doctor, The American Heart Association, The American Stroke Association, or other excellent informational sources. *(see Page 150 for some websites.)*

HEART

♥	Fist-sized blood-pumping organ	(heart)
♥	Essence	(heart of the matter)
♥	Core	(heart of the earth)
♥	Conscience	(heart won't let me)
♥	Love	(give you my heart)
♥	Devotion	(from bottom of my heart)
♥	Determination	(heart to go on)
♥	Sympathy	(heart goes out to you)
♥	Bad Feeling	(heavy heart)
♥	Good Feeling	(light-hearted)
♥	Courage	(brave heart)
♥	Valentine	(paper heart)
♥	Smitten	(stole my heart)
♥	Fundamental	(heart of the matter)
♥	Memorize	(learn by heart)
♥	Knowledge	(in my heart I know)
♥	Encouragement	(take heart)
♥	Absolute Truth	(cross my heart)
♥	Kindness	(have a heart)
♥	Best Part	(heart of watermelon)
♥	Compassion	(have a heart for)
♥	Spirit	(broken heart)
♥	Dedication	(heart isn't in it)
♥	Very Most Basic	(heart of hearts)
♥	Playing Card	(Queen of Hearts)
♥	Favorite Piano Duet	(Heart & Soul)
♥	Conviction	(with all my heart)

13
Estrogen and Osteoporosis

METABOLISM

Metabolism is a broad term describing the chemical processes going on inside our body. There are two types of metabolism. A **catabolic** process is the chemical process that breaks down a substance for use. An **anabolic** process is the chemical process that builds up a substance for use. Hormones control most metabolic activity, and when there is an under-production or overproduction of a hormone, the chemical process will not function correctly. Estrogen is one of the primary hormones that helps maintain our metabolism. When estrogen decreases, body tissue breaks down faster than it can re-form. This is the root cause of problems encountered by menopausal women such as osteoporosis, muscle thinning, and weight retention.

OSTEOPOROSIS *OSTEO (Bone) POROSIS (porous)*

Estrogen helps keep calcium in the bones. As the amount of estrogen is decreased, bones lose **collagen**, taking calcium with it. This causes bones to be less dense which makes them become brittle and weak. This is osteoporosis. Both hard and spongy bone tissue are affected.

Half of all women will experience osteoporosis to some degree.

Osteoporosis is a gradual disease. Although most bone density is lost during the first 2-5 years of menopause, it is over the next 10-15 years that osteoporosis actually develops. It is called a silent disease because there are no warning signals. Early signs of osteoporosis may be backaches. Later, bones may fracture more easily. The skeletal damage that occurs when vertebrae become weak and then collapse can cause older people to lose several inches in height. *Dowager's hump* and loss of height are symptoms of advanced osteoporosis. Besides the characteristic "hump" or rounded back, curvature of the spine can lead to nerve damage resulting in pain. As bones thin, vertebral fractures can occur merely by coughing or bending. Most commonly, bone fractures, especially of the hip, are responsible for loss of mobility and even premature death.

RISK FACTORS

Besides being of menopausal age and experiencing estrogen loss, there are other high risk factors. Among these are being Caucasian or Asian, having a slender body build, a family history of osteoporosis, or entering menopause before age 45 due to non-natural menopause such as surgery. You may also be at a higher risk if you smoke, drink alcohol, don't exercise, and don't get enough calcium and Vitamin D in your diet. Women who do not menstruate, especially because of eating disorders like anorexia nervosa, are at risk. Also at risk are persons using thyroid drugs, prednisone or other corticosteroid drugs which interfere with calcium regulation and the cells that maintain bones, resulting in brittle bones. (The thyroid controls metabolic rates and levels of calcium in the blood.) Also, diseases like Type I diabetes and rheumatoid arthritis disrupt the body's ability to build and retain bone. As men age, testosterone levels can decrease which contributes to osteoporosis in men, too. (see Chapter 23)

DEXA

Other than an unexpected bone fracture, there are few ways to know when bones are becoming less dense. One of the best means to detect loss of bone mass is through imaging or x-ray. Currently, the best diagnostic tool is Dual Energy X-Ray Absorptiometry (DEXA or DXA) which is a low-level x-ray that measures bone density in the hips and lower spine. Also available is a heel ultrasound which isn't as accurate as DEXA but is faster, less expensive and a good screener to see if DEXA is needed.

HRT, CALCIUM and EXERCISE

There is discussion concerning reversing the effects of osteoporosis using diet, exercise, calcium supplements, and hormone replacement therapy. It is believed that most bone growth happens up to age 25. After this age, it is important to maintain what bone we have and try to prevent loss of bone mass.

CALCIUM

Calcium is the mineral most often associated with bone. Remember when your mom told you to drink your milk so that when you grew up you would have strong bones and teeth. Well, she was right. As mentioned, it is believed that most bone growth happens before we're out of high school. Between then and when we enter the menopausal stages, calcium is pretty much maintained. However, once estrogen production begins to fade, bone calcium may begin to leech out. So can just taking more calcium replace all that bone mass? Probably not. What it can do, however, is keep any more from leaving.

Proper calcium intake throughout our life is a key way to prevent osteoporosis. Unfortunately, most females of all ages do not get enough calcium. Milk, of course, is the best source of nutritional calcium. But it is not a consistent part of the average diet. Perhaps because of lactose intolerance or calorie avoidance. But, primarily, because in a world revolving around fast food, we just don't include many calcium-rich foods in our diet. Let's look at some of these.

DIETARY SOURCES of CALCIUM

Excellent sources of dietary calcium are the many products made from soy, such as milk, yogurt, tofu, beans, & nuts. Other good sources are broccoli, figs, dark-green leafy vegetables like spinach, kale, and collard and turnip greens, rice milk, canned sardines and salmon, almonds and other nuts, and cheeses like mozzarella and cheddar. Additional good sources are foods with added calcium like some cereals and breads, instant oatmeal, and juices like cranberry and orange juice. In some cases, these fortified foods supply more calcium than milk!

CALCIUM SUPPLEMENTS

Since we're probably not going to eat enough calcium-rich foods, the next best thing is to take a good calcium supplement. But how much? Which ones?

DOSAGE

Dosages vary depending on your lifestyle, diet, and whether or not you're taking HRT. Even though calcium supplements are sold without a prescription, it's a good idea to discuss them with your doctor.

A general dosage suggestion is:

Women ages 25-50	500-800 mg daily
Post-menopausal women	800-1500 mg daily

Unless under a doctor's care, most sources suggest not taking more than 1500 mg per day of calcium. Also, since the body can only absorb small amounts of calcium at a time, the above amounts should be taken with half in the morning and half later in the day.

CALCIUM PARTNERS

As with all the components in our body, calcium doesn't work alone. Calcium is best absorbed when properly balanced with other minerals such as **Vitamins C and D**, **magnesium**, **manganese**, **zinc**, and **copper**. A good multiple vitamin and mineral supplement will usually have a correct balance of these nutrients. The National Osteoporosis Foundation has a general recommendation of 1500 mg calcium, 600 mg magnesium, and 400 mg Vit. D daily. Check with your doctor.

There are both good and bad interactions of calcium with other foods. In a positive way, **Vitamin D** doubles calcium absorption which is why it is often added to milk. **Vitamin C** improves absorption of calcium carbonate so it is best taken with orange, grapefruit, or cranberry juices. In a negative way, high amounts of **phosphorus** cause a mineral imbalance which interferes with proper calcium absorption. Soft drinks are particularly high in phosphoric acid, as are many canned foods. **Caffeine** "binds" calcium and limits its absorption. Caffeine is a natural diuretic and can cause too much calcium to be washed out of our system. Caffeine also washes out other minerals important for calcium absorption. **Alcoholic drinks** have the same diuretic effect.

CALCIUM CITRATE/CALCIUM CARBONATE

There are a number of types of calcium supplements. **Calcium citrate** and **calcium carbonate** are two popular choices. Calcium carbonate is best absorbed after meals while calcium citrate works any time. Read the information provided by the manufacturer or talk with your doctor to determine which supplement is best for you.

Blood tests may determine that you have too much or too little calcium in your bloodstream. Both conditions need attention. Too much calcium in your blood might sound like calcium overload but may actually mean a calcium deficiency due to an inefficient utilization of calcium by your body. There are also times when you may need prescription medications to enhance calcium absorption.

HRT and OSTEOPOROSIS

Estrogen replacement therapy slows bone loss. **Statins** (drugs used to reduce cholesterol levels and prevent heart disease) may also reduce the risk of osteoporosis although they do have side effects. (Your doctor will explain these.)

WEIGHT-BEARING EXERCISE

Calcium supplements and even estrogen replacement may not replace bone loss that has already occurred although they may stop further bone loss. Weight-bearing exercises, however, may stop bone loss and actually rebuild bone. Weight lifting, particularly in combination with calcium intake, may reverse osteoporosis by building new bone and increasing bone density. In addition to strengthening bone, weight-bearing exercise replenishes the *synovial fluid* that lubricates joints and prevents stiffness. (Synovial fluid is a clear, sticky fluid secreted by the membranes of movable joint areas which provides lubrication for those joints.)

Weight-bearing exercises are exactly what their name imply. When you walk or jog, your legs, hips, spine, etc. are bearing the full weight of your body. Lifting weight with your arms or legs is considered a weight-bearing exercise. When body muscles are stimulated, that action then stimulates bones in that area. For full benefit, try to **exercise** your entire body. You may discuss with your doctor any exercise program to fit your personal physical condition. You can vary your weight-bearing exercise routine by also including hiking, skiing, aerobic dancing and stair climbing. Unless you're already proficient in weight-lifting, here are some general recommendations for weight-bearing exercises.

Use 2-5 pounds for upper body muscles. Try 30-minutes of weight-lifting, twice a week, exercising all your body areas. To increase bone density in hips and legs, walk briskly 30 minutes, 3 times a week. (Check with your doctor before embarking on any exercise program.)

Heartburn?

Don't forget that some popular antacids supply a hefty amount of calcium carbonate. Check the label.

14
Estrogen and Other Things It Messes Up

BREAST TENDERNESS

Estrogen causes breast cells to retain excess fluid which results in fullness and tenderness, especially around menstruation and when using hormone replacement therapy.

EYES

Researchers are looking at a likely connection between estrogen loss and three eye disorders: *macular degeneration, cataracts,* and *glaucoma.* Indications are that twice as many older women develop macular degeneration as older men, leading researchers to strongly believe that this is a result of estrogen loss. Although about the same number of women as men develop cataracts, there is strong evidence that a woman's chance of getting cataracts drops in correlation with the number of years she has natural estrogen or she takes a hormone replacement. There may also a connection between estrogen and the fluid retention in the eye leading to glaucoma. Researchers are still trying to figure out if the culprit is estrogen, progesterone, or a combination of the two. See your eye doctor for complete information and regular eye examinations.

Macular degeneration is a progressive disorder in which the central part of the retina is gradually blocked by scar tissue, a result of fluid leakage in the layers of the eye. The result is rarely total blindness.

The person retains peripheral (side) vision although they lose their central vision. (It looks like a big thumbprint right in center of their field of vision.)

Cataracts develop when the lens of the eye becomes clouded due to changes in the protein fibers in the eye. (Similar to what happens to the white of an egg when it is cooked.) Cataracts do not cause total blindness and are now easily removed surgically.

Glaucoma is a condition in which the fluids in the eye build up too much pressure and damage the nerve fibers. Complete or partial blindness can result.

FACIAL HAIR GROWTH

Each month, the ovaries release estrogen and progesterone into the blood stream. They also release a small amount of **testosterone** (one of the androgen hormones.) Prior to menopause, this small amount of testosterone, the hormone that produces male characteristics, has been counterbalanced by the estrogen. After menopause, when estrogen production becomes irregular, the testosterone goes unchecked and can cause male traits like facial hair, which usually appears on the upper lip or chin. Estrogen replacement will stop more hair from growing but won't get rid of hair that's already grown.

FACIAL PIGMENTATION CHANGES

One of the less common side effects of hormone changes is facial pigmentation. Common or not, the appearance of sudden dark splotches on a woman's face is nothing to take lightly. Estrogen, along with **MSH (Melanocyte-stimulating hormone),** stimulates pigmentation in nipples and may be responsible for causing a darkening of facial skin. Although this is most often associated with pregnancy and is even called the Mask of Pregnancy, it can also occur in menopausal women or women taking oral contraceptives. The medical term is **Chloasma** or **Melasma**.

It is characterized by blotches of pale, green-brown skin pigmentation that occur on the forehead, cheeks, and nose. When there are so many of these dark blotches that they "merge", it is called a **mask**. The change in pigmentation is aggravated by sunlight so direct sunlight should be avoided when this condition is present. When hormone levels are again balanced, the blotches usually fade, although in some cases the condition may be permanent. In women of child-bearing age, becoming pregnant again may cause this pigmentation to recur.

GALLSTONES

There appears to be a connection between estrogen and the development of gallstones. This has to do with the correlation between estrogen, cholesterol and metabolism. **Metabolism** is a broad term describing the chemical processes going on inside our body that involve either breaking down or building up a substance for use. The proper flow of estrogen is vital for proper metabolism. It is also vital for controlling the amount of good and bad cholesterol in the body. The **liver** is the central chemical processing plant for the body. Among its many jobs, the liver produces **cholesterol**, and it produces bile. **Bile** carries waste products away from the liver and helps in the breakdown and absorption of fats. It is stored in a little sac under the liver called the **gallbladder**. Cholesterol is vital for a properly functioning body, but it has gotten a bad reputation because there is often too much bad cholesterol and not enough good. **Gallstones** are primarily composed of cholesterol. When the bile is overloaded with cholesterol, a tiny solid particle can form that may grow as more and more materials solidify around it. Just as cholesterol plaque can cause clogs in the bloodstream, gallstones can clog ducts around the gallbladder. Because of the hormonal connection between estrogen and metabolism, it is not surprising that women have more than twice the number of gallstones as men. Also because of the hormonal effect, women who have used birth control pills or who take estrogen replacement therapy are at a higher risk for developing gallstones. Other risk factors are being overweight and women who have had many children (both are connected with changes in metabolism.) Although as we get older most people have gallstones, the person is often unaware they have them unless they cause problems. To prevent gallstones, do not become overweight, avoid HRT, and avoid a diet high in fat and sugars.

GINGIVITIS

In the dental world, it is known that pregnant women may experience what is called **pregnant** or **gestational gingivitis. Plaque** is a sticky accumulation of food particles, saliva, and bacteria that builds up on teeth near the gumline and can cause gums to bleed or become inflamed. This plaque build-up appears to happen more frequently in pregnant women due to increased hormone levels. A similar phenomenon may occur in menopausal women when there are also hormonal imbalances. (Hormones do not cause the gingivitis. They just seem to exaggerate how the plaque irritates the gums.) As always, you should maintain good oral health and dental care. Your dentist can more fully explain the connection between estrogen imbalances and gingivitis.

HEADACHES AND MIGRAINES

Estrogen fluctuations may be connected to headaches and migraine headaches. Pre-menopausal women who experience migraines usually develop them 1-2 days before their period begins and into the first two days of their period. This is linked to the fall of estrogen. This same decrease in estrogen makes menopausal women susceptible to migraines or regular headaches.

Pre-menopausal women are often given the estrogen patch during these 5 days to ease migraines. The same may work for menopausal sufferers.

HEARING

Not only that, but hormonal changes appear to be responsible for some hearing loss in menopausal women. The hormonal changes appear to diminish blood flow to the structures in the ear that affect hearing loss, particularly at low frequencies. Men start losing hearing first. After age 50, men hear lower level sounds better than higher levels but, after menopause, women can't hear lower level sounds any better than men can. Menopausal women may also have difficulty hearing more than one sound at a time which prevents them from detecting tone nuances like humor or sarcasm. (FYI: The right hemisphere of the brain controls voice cues.) Usually after age 70, when hormones finally stop fluctuating, these hearing disturbances seem to diminish. It's always been known that hearing is affected by exposure to sounds, genetics, gender and injury. It now appears that hormones affect hearing, too.

TEETH

In addition to gingivitis, estrogen declines can also cause tooth loss. Jawbones are subject to the same loss of density as other bones in the body, and teeth can come out when jawbones become too weak to hold them in place. (This is the same principle discussed in Chapter 13.)

15
Estrogen and Memory

Right after *Is it hot in here? Or is it just me?* the second most common phrase uttered by menopausal women is *I can't remember anything any more.* Estrogen fluctuations are to blame again! Estrogen helps to maintain the brain's "memory bank." This is because estrogen affects the **hippocampus** which is a part of the brain most involved with memory functions. When estrogen levels are high, the brain can take in more information. That's because estrogen is believed to protect brain cells by activating the parts of the brain used to store information. Estrogen may also shield the brain cells from wear and tear, stimulate nerve growth, and increase blood flow to the brain. Estrogen has been proven to be vital in the proper functioning of the memory process and may also help build new circuits in the brain.

Estrogen levels can begin to dip as early as age 35 although it mostly happens in the 40's and 50's. Not coincidentally, this is when many women start experiencing problems with memory. Estrogen appears to primarily affect short term memory. That's why we can remember the color of our Sunday School teacher's favorite dress but can't remember what we had for dinner yesterday. As men age and lose testosterone, they have memory loss, too, although it appears that the brain cells of post-menopausal women degenerate at a faster pace than men of the same age, which is responsible, in part, for the higher incidence of Alzheimer's in women than in men. The loss of sleep due to night sweats may also greatly affect memory as sleep deprivation is often a cause of memory impairment.

HRT and MEMORY

Hormone Replacement Therapy has been proven to help with memory loss in menopausal women. Women who take HRT seem to have improved memory and reasoning skills. Using the diagnostic tool MRI, women taking estrogen appear to show more activity in brain areas associated with memory retrieval and encoding. Many studies suggest that estrogen replacement can slash the chance of Alzheimer's. In other studies, women who used estrogen replacement therapy had better short term memory; for example, remembering phone numbers they had just looked up.

MEMORY TRICKS and TOOLS

If you do not use HRT, there are ways to deal with this memory impairment. Let those little yellow **sticky-notes** become your best friend. Keep pads everywhere you might need to jot down something, even in your car. Hang an erasable board on the refrigerator, near your desk, or wherever you need one. If you can't trust your memory, learn to **write it down**! (Of course, you'll have to remember where you put all those little notes!) **Rhymes** and **mnemonic devices** (nee MON ick) are neat memory tools. (Remember, in grade school we learned the little rhyme, "In 14 hundred and 92, Columbus sailed the ocean blue.") So are **associational tricks**. If the letters of your license plate are 747 CNC, you might picture a jet landing in Charlotte, North Carolina. The idea is to associate something familiar or firmly engrained in your memory with something that isn't so firmly engrained.

Memory Retention?
The only thing I retain is water!

16
Estrogen and Hot Flashes and Night Sweats

So where were you when you first uttered those immortal words, "Is it hot in here? Or is it just me?" Probably nothing is more associated with menopause than hot flashes. Jokes are made about them, but any woman will tell you that they're no laughing matter. So let's look at hot flashes and their partner in crime, night sweats.

HOT FLASHES

So what exactly is a hot flash? Back to biology. The autonomic nervous system affects the controlled **dilation** (opening) and **constriction** (closing) of the tiny blood vessels in muscles and skin called capillaries. This means that your system automatically tells the blood vessels in your muscles and skin when to open and close to keep your body perfectly climate-controlled. These are called **vasomotor** functions (*Vaso* means *vessel,* which in this case refers to blood vessels.) The vasomotor function regulates the size of the blood vessels by making them constrict or dilate. In **vasoconstriction,** the body senses "cold" on the skin. To maintain a constant body temperature, the blood vessels narrow, reducing blood flow, which reduces the body's heat loss. **Vasodilatation** is just the opposite. When the skin feels hot, the vessels widen. Blood flow is increased, which makes us sweat, and sweat accelerates heat loss from the body. As the body sweats to keep cool, the dilation also causes **flushing**.

This flushing is a wave of heat and perspiring, maybe even accompanied by a redness of the skin.

This flush is the same sensation experienced by menopausal women, but for different reasons. Rather than being stimulated by a sensation of hot or cold, estrogen fluctuations cause the capillaries to rapidly open and then close just as fast. When opened, a rush of blood causes the hot flash. When suddenly closed, a chill-down occurs. Flushes usually last only several minutes although they may occur repeatedly throughout the day. These hot flashes begin in perimenopause and continue far past the actual cessation of periods. Because of the similarity to the word flush, and because these waves come and go so quickly (in a *flash*, you might say), this thoroughly annoying experience is what we know as a **hot flash**.

The wave of heat starts at the top of your head and goes all the way to your feet. But it seems that certain areas get "hotter" than others. Your forehead, chest area, the bends at the knees and elbows, your neck, and the bottoms of your feet get really hot. Your shins won't get hot, but your thighs will feel like they're being smothered.

The average person has 3 million sweat glands.

CHILL-DOWN

Not only will you get unbearably hot when the flush occurs, but when it suddenly goes away, you will often be chilled to the bone. That's perfectly understandable when you consider that sweat on the skin is a natural air conditioner. But it doesn't make it any easier to take. No wonder we get irritable. Chill-downs can be as bothersome as hot flashes.

SURVIVING HOT FLASHES

Dealing with hot flashes is not easy. Hormone Replacement Therapy will pretty much take care of hot flashes and night sweats. But for women who want to avoid the side effects associated with **HRT**, there are options. Some **herbal products** may help, and these are discussed in Chapter 19.

Unless you opt for HRT, you're just going to have to sweat (ha!) it out until the estrogen fluctuations start to go away. (This will only take, say, ten or fifteen years!) A little common sense goes a long way here. Let's start first with **room temperature**. Before you waltz over to the thermostat to adjust it AGAIN, see what it actually reads. If it says 70 degrees but you're sweltering, it's a hot flash. If it says 77 degrees, it's not you. It IS hot in the room. Then it's safe to make a thermostat adjustment. Even though you may be sweating your socks off, followed up by a major chill-down, please don't make everyone else around you miserable by constantly adjusting the thermostat or opening/closing windows.

Your best bet is to invest in **fans**. Put one in every room so you can turn it on whenever you need a quick cool-off. Since they're small, you can turn a fan directly on you and not upset the rest of the gang. Plus, they're cheap to purchase and cost next to nothing to operate. Set a small oscillating fan on your chest of drawers. An even-smaller model works great on the bathroom vanity or on the kitchen countertop. There are even tiny hand-held, battery-powered models for taking with you. Not to mention ones that hook into an automobile's cigarette lighter that can be angled directly at you for those hot flashes in the car. (It beats rolling down the window and hanging out your head like a beagle!)

NIGHT SWEATS

Night sweats are nothing more than hot flashes that happen at night. But, because at night we're usually wrapped up in blankets and pajamas, the effect seems worse than during the day. Many of us sleep in the fetal position at least part of the night. All curled up like that, the chest and neck areas get the hottest because all that heat is trapped between our arms and breasts. The back of the head, where it rests against the pillow, is hot to the touch. Where we're lying on the bed will be hot, too, or even wet with perspiration. Plus, there is the restlessness caused by feet that are cold as ice on top and burning up on the bottoms. When sleep finally does come, it's interrupted throughout the night when we wake up clammy, often soaking in our own perspiration. When that passes, we're chilled.

You wake up comfortable. Then you roll over.
All of a sudden, you're sweating bullets.
Rolling over just isn't that much of a strenuous activity.
Night sweats!

SURVIVING NIGHT SWEATS

For women who forego HRT and choose to go through the Change cold turkey, night sweats can be the worst part of all the menopausal symptoms. More than one woman has sat on the edge of the bed or sofa crying, desperate for some sleep but too miserably hot and sweaty to get any. Since HRT may only ease these symptoms, not make them go away entirely, there are some non-medicinal tricks to get through these night sweats. The most obvious is to be sure the **room temperature** is actually not too hot. Sometimes the action of a heater or a/c cycling on and off throughout the night disrupts a uniform temperature. Although it sounds contradictory, some women have found that turning the room temperature up a little and then sleeping under a fan works best because the fan blows a consistent temperature of air on them rather than the on and off action of the a/c or furnace.

Now that menopause has changed everything, you may find you start wearing different types of **sleeping garments**. It seems that most women sleep better if they are evenly dressed from head to toe. That may even mean wearing socks, even if you never wore them to bed before.

When you wake up hot and sweaty, the first thing you might do is **roll over** on your back. This will help the heat escape from your chest area.

Silly as it seems, another thing guaranteed to keep you awake and dealing with night sweats is the need to **go to the bathroom**. Even though it's thoroughly aggravating, try getting on up and going to the bathroom each time you are awakened. More than one woman has declared that if she'll just get up and go to the bathroom the minute she awakens, she can come back to bed and sleep. If she lies there without getting up, she'll sweat and sweat, and toss and turn. Plus, moving around cools you off some and allows the bedding to cool, too.

Keeping your body against **cool sheets** works wonders, even if you have to keep flipping from one side of the bed to another. Don't forget to flip your pillow, too. The underside of a pillowcase can be wonderfully cool against a hot, sweaty head. If you have a mattress that can be climate-controlled, take advantage of that feature.

IT'S JUST TEMPORARY, HONEY

For married women, you may have to sleep in the spare bedroom or on the sofa occasionally. If you're sweating profusely, neither you nor your husband will get any sleep if you spend most of the night kicking off blankets and then pulling them back on. You need to be able to flip from one side of the bed to the other in your search for cool sheets, and you can't do that if he's taking up half the bed. Since temporarily changing your sleeping arrangements might be a touchy subject, talk it out with your husband. (see Chapter 24) It's not a permanent situation. Just a way to get some sleep...for both of you.

Hot flashes are pesky, but do not fret....
no one's ever drowned in sweat.

17
Estrogen and Emotions

PSYCHOLOGICAL ISSUES

Sometimes the hormonal fluctuations in a woman's body are nothing compared with the emotional upheavals going on at the same time caused by either menopausal effects or a culmination of life experiences. When a woman reaches her 40's and 50's, there's a lot more changing than just estrogen flow.

Estrogen does create a lot of emotional concerns. As it decreases, we may have trouble concentrating, remembering, and even making decisions. The lack of sleep associated with night sweats compounds these, and a whole lot more. When we don't get enough sleep, we get cranky, easily fatigued, and tearful. This can make us tense. Emotional tension can cause muscle spasms, even in the heart muscle. We may develop little twitches in our eye or above the upper lip. The excessive emotional tension can cause hyperventilation which makes us short of breath and makes our arms and feet tingle and feel kind of numb. Those sensations can bring on fears of heart attack or stroke. As hormone fluctuations vary and affect the brain, our moods can change. The same hormone variances that cause pregnant women to be lethargic, depressed or easily angered are responsible for the same symptoms in menopausal women. As hormones ebb and flow, a woman can actually feel a wave of sadness come over her. And she is aware that's she's being annoyed, if not enraged, at things that never used to rile her at all.

FULL BUCKET

But there can be a lot more that makes us cry or get frustrated than just hormone changes. Menopause is often just the last drop that makes our bucket overflow. Look at what may have been filling that bucket over 45-50 years of life. Career pressures, kids, PTA, divorce, financial worries, in-law problems, illnesses, mortgages, lost friendships, the declining health or death of parents, taxes, and the look-in-the-mirror confirmation that we're not as young as we used to be. We are woman, wife, breadwinner, bread cooker, mother, grandmother, aunt, daughter, caregiver, shopper, accountant, nurse, chauffeur, psychologist, teacher, disciplinarian, and general jack-of-all trades. A full bucket, indeed!

LOSS OF ABILITY TO BEAR CHILDREN

The assumed loss of womanhood is a real problem for a lot of women. Just as their kids are leaving home and the empty-nest syndrome is kicking in, along comes menopause. An in-your-face declaration that you can no longer bear children. Nothing characterizes womanhood more than the ability to have kids. And now, because of menopause, it's gone. For women who have always wanted kids but never had them, this is particularly hard. For women who have born children, it's still hard. It's like something that is so inherently *US* is gone.

LOSS OF BODY PARTS

Women who undergo a mastectomy or hysterectomy have to deal with the physical loss of a part of their sexuality. For some women, this is a serious issue. As with any loss, the woman may have to go through some kind of grieving process. For other women, it's simply a hunk of tissue that is only a part of her physical body. She is far more than a breast or uterus. They are just a part of her physical body. It is not her identity. Many women are worried that their husband will find them less sexual. This is rarely an issue for a caring man. When a man and woman have shared a loving relationship, their sexuality is MUCH more than skin deep.

EMOTIONAL INSTABILITY

For a time, while this menopause thing is raging alongside all our Life Experiences, we may actually find ourselves being a little emotionally unstable. Not because we're nuts. But because there's just a lot going on, externally and internally. But it's only temporary. As the hormones stop wildly fluctuating, we are able to get a grip on things again. Eventually this wildest of all roller coaster rides does come to an end. There are helpful ways to get through this period.

Most importantly, realize this is only a temporary state of affairs. Learn to deal with your emotions. We can't make them go away, but we can make some conscious decisions about how we're going to handle them. You can decide to be tearful rather than hateful. This is not to say that you will never be hateful or fly off the handle. Just TRY not to do those things. Some women know they are being nasty and do it anyway, just writing their bad behavior off on menopause. That's probably not a good idea. There's no reason to make everyone else pay for your hormonal changes.

Misery may love company
but company does NOT love misery.

RELIEF

Some women find relief by taking a shower or long bath. There is something soothing about the feel of **water on your skin** and how it symbolically washes away what's ailing us. Take as many a day as makes you feel comfortable. Worry about the water bill later. Some have an **anger room** where they bang the closet door for a while or beat a hammer on a piece of wood. (Be kind of careful with this one because sometimes being angry just makes you angrier.) Some women excuse themselves for a **good cry** when they feel one coming on. If you start hyperventilating, puffing, or twitching, **decompress** by reading or simply lying down. Others go for a walk or run. **Physical exercise** is great for tension release because it relaxes muscle spasms and contributes to the release of "feel-good" endorphins. Take a **nap** if you are becoming sleep deprived. Maybe it's time to **learn** something new. **Get creative** with a hobby or interest like painting or crafts. **Get involved** in your community or church by volunteering. Turn your spare bedroom into a room devoted to YOUR special interests. **Travel**.

Enjoy life!

REALITY CHECK

You ARE going to have wild swings in your emotions. You ARE going to find yourself more sentimental. You ARE going to explode in rage at the clown with 50 items in the express lane. You ARE going to be sitting innocently on the sofa and feel a wave of sadness start at the top of your head and wash all the way down to your toes. You ARE going to be weirdly moody. You ARE going to cry buckets at a broken fingernail. You ARE going to have **panic attacks** and feel like you're going to crawl out of your skin.

Expect these and prepare for how you're going to deal with them. Do not be afraid to ask for help during emotionally or physically rough times. You probably don't have to run to a counselor, but it's plenty OK to talk to your family about how you're feeling. If you need some help around the house, tell someone. If you're tired of doing something just because you've always done it, stop. You've been the support system for nearly everyone in your life up until now. It's OK to do a little leaning once in a while. (By the way, do seek professional help if you think it's necessary.)

HRT and OTHER REMEDIES

The estrogen part of hormone replacement therapy will usually level off your emotions, and some herbal products can be soothing and act like natural tranquilizers. (see Chapters 18 and 19)

18
Hormone Replacement Therapy
Prescription Products

HORMONE REPLACEMENT THERAPY (HRT)

Depending with whom you talk, HRT can either stand for *Heart* (*we love it*) or *Hurt* (*we don't like it at all.*) Hormone replacement therapy is a hotly debated discussion. Do the positives outweigh the negatives? How can there be bad side effects by simply replacing what was naturally occurring in our body? Let's take a look at HRT. Although there are a myriad of hormones that can be used in hormone replacement therapies, the ones associated with menopause are **estrogen** and **progesterone**. They may be used separately or in tandem to treat symptoms of the Change or to prevent conditions associated with the loss of our female hormones. In some discussions, you may find distinct references to **estrogen replacement therapy** (**ERT**.) However in most discussions, estrogen replacement is not differentiated but is referred to, alone or in combination with progesterone, as HRT. Whenever HRT is mentioned in the *Menopause Survival Guide,* it refers to any hormone replacement therapy, alone or with another hormone.

CAUTION

When taking replacement hormones, it's always best to start with low doses and work up rather than the other way around. There are many drugs from which to choose, and you should work closely with your doctor to find the one that works best for you. Since during the perimenopausal stage there is a chance of **pregnancy**, do not take any hormone therapy if you are pregnant or could get pregnant. As with all medications, keep them out of the reach of children and pets. There have been some cases of small children developing enlarged breasts and other feminine traits because they have either handled an estrogen patch or come in repeated contact with an estrogen cream. All discarded estrogen patches should be carefully disposed of, and hands should be thoroughly washed after applying estrogen cream and before touching children. Treat these drugs as you would all drugs and **keep them out of the reach of children**.

Make your own decisions about hormone replacement therapy. You will be bombarded with ads on TV, in magazines, and in brochures in the doctor's office promoting a manufacturer's drugs. They want you to buy their products. Be a wise consumer. Buy it if you need it. Don't buy it if you don't need it or don't want it.

SIDE EFFECTS

Whether you're considering prescription or over-the-counter remedies, be aware of all the side effects of hormone replacement therapy. Everything seems to have a pro and con. *One woman took combined estrogen and progesterone hormone replacement. It worked great on her hot flashes and night sweats. However, it also caused her periods to resume. At age 65, she definitely did NOT want that!* So she went back to her doctor, discussed her concerns with him, and they made adjustments in her medication.

Because of information in the previous chapters of the *Menopause Survival Guide*, as you look through the Positives and Negatives lists, you will be able to understand how hormone replacement can affect your body. In the case of some medications that have not been previously discussed, they are briefly explained at the end of this chapter. PLEASE discuss side effects and drug interactions with your doctor.

COMBINED ESTROGENS

EQUINE URINE-BASED ESTROGENS

Our body naturally makes a combination of estrogens (estradiol, estriol, and estrone.) Replacement estrogen products are also a combination of estrogens. They are called **conjugated** (combined) estrogens. Nearly all estrogen replacement drugs are made from combined estrogens taken from the **urine of pregnant horses.** (You may also see them called *conjugated equine estrogens. Equine*, of course, relates to horses.) The urine is collected from mares, and the estrogens are chemically separated from the urine. These estrogens are then "put together" in a process called synthesis. The result is a synthetic conjugated estrogen hormone product. The best known estrogen drug is **Premarin** (Wyeth-Ayerst.) PRE (*pregnant*) MAR(*mare*) IN (*urine*). Many other companies make estrogen replacements, of course. Consult your doctor, pharmacist or the drug manufacturer for information about benefits and side effects.

Conjugated estrogens, derived from the urine of pregnant mares, were first approved by the FDA in 1938.

PLANT-BASED ESTROGENS

Although urine-based estrogen products are the most widely prescribed, some **plant-based** estrogens have also been produced. In 1999, the FDA approved **Cenestin** as a prescription medication to treat hot flashes and night sweats but not for long-term use such as helping prevent osteoporosis. Cenestin is a conjugated estrogen made from nine synthetic estrogen components which are chemically derived from compounds found in some plants. As above, contact your doctor or the manufacturer (Duramed) for more information.

The following information concerns estrogen products made from pregnant mare urine, not plant estrogens.

ESTROGEN

Positives for Estrogen Replacement Therapy

- Increases bone mineral density.
- Reduces risk of bone fractures from osteoporosis.
- May reduce some risk of heart disease.
- May lower incidence of stroke, colon and ovarian cancer, and diabetes.
- May lower incidence of blindness due to cataracts and macular degeneration.
- Keeps skin younger looking and less dry, and lowers incidence of tooth and hair loss.
- May lower overall mortality.
- Possibly lowers chance of developing Alzheimer's.
- Keeps cholesterol in check by elevating good cholesterol.

Negatives for Estrogen Replacement Therapy

- Estrogen alone increases the risk of breast cancer.
- Estrogen alone causes an overgrowth in the uterine lining which may lead to uterine cancer.
- May increase risk of heart attack in the first year for women with coronary artery disease. (Often because HRT is administered in dosages too high.)
- Causes breast tenderness and enlargement.
- Causes bloating, weight gain, nausea, vomiting, abdominal cramps and vaginal bleeding.

- May cause loss of scalp hair.
- Promotes gallstones and gall bladder disease.
- Creates reduced sex drive and depression.
- May cause spasms of arteries that cause migraines and headaches.
- May increase risk of hypertension (high blood pressure.)
- Estrogen increases the possibility of abnormal blood clotting. (Not recommended for women with personal or family history of heart disease, stroke, pulmonary embolism or deep-vein thrombosis.)
- May cause problems with blood clotting so should not be taken by women about to undergo surgery.
- May interact with smoking tobacco. The AMA has warned that smoking tobacco while taking estrogen drugs significantly increases the risk of abnormal blood clotting which may cause myocardial infarction, pulmonary embolism or stroke.
- May interact with corticosteroids, oral blood thinners, barbiturates, tamoxifen and tricyclic anti-depressants. (See the end of this chapter.)
- Not recommended for women with heavy vaginal bleeding, circulation problems or history of breast cancer.

PROGESTERONE

Progesterone used in hormone replacement therapy is derived primarily from wild yams which contain a compound called *diosgenin.* Within the composition of diosgenin is a molecule of progesterone that can be separated from the rest of the diosgenin in a laboratory. This fragment is the basis for replacement progesterone. (Major drug companies operate huge farms where wild yams are grown.) The technical term for the progesterone replacement hormone is *medroxy-*

progesterone, and synthetic progesterones are called *progestins*. For menopausal women, progesterone replacement is used primarily to reduce the risk of uterine cancer. Progesterone may be administered by tablet, injection or cream. Although it is not the only product, a well-known progesterone replacement is **Provera** (Upjohn.) Consult your doctor, pharmacist or the manufacturer for information about benefits and side effects.

The first synthetic progesterone appeared in the 1940's.

Positives for Progesterone Replacement Therapy

- Reduces risk of uterine cancer associated with estrogen therapy.
- Treats endometriosis and endometrial cancer by preventing overgrowth of uterine lining.
- Treats symptoms associated with PMS.
- Helps underdeveloped ovaries.
- Effective means of birth control.
  - Alters cervical mucous so sperm cannot penetrate it.
  - Alters uterine lining so that fertilized egg cannot attach to lining and grow.
  - Reduces hormone production that makes egg ripen in the ovary.

Negatives for Progesterone Replacement Therapy

- May cause weight gain or loss of appetite.
- May cause rash or edema.
- May cause headache or dizziness.
- May cause irregular periods.
- May cause breast tenderness.
- May cause ovarian cysts.

ESTROGEN and PROGESTERONE COMBINED

Conjugated estrogens and medroxyprogesterone are often prescribed to more closely resemble natural hormone production in the female body. A well-known combination drug is **PremPro** (Wyeth-Ayerst.) PremPro is made of conjugated estrogens and medroxy-progesterone acetate. Contact your doctor, pharmacist or the manufacturer for information about benefits and side effects.

Positives for Combined Estrogen/Progesterone Hormone Replacement Therapy

- Provides benefits associated with estrogen therapy.
- Reduces risk of uterine cancer associated with overgrowth of the uterine lining linked with estrogen therapy.

Negatives for Combined Estrogen/Progesterone Hormone Replacement Therapy

- May cause breast enlargement, pain or tenderness.
- May cause headache and fatigue.
- May cause nausea, vomiting, abdominal cramps, vaginal bleeding or discharge.
- May interact with corticosteroids, warfarin, barbiturates, and tricyclic antidepressants. (See end of this chapter.)
- Not recommended for women with unusual vaginal bleeding or circulation problems.
- Not recommended for women with history of breast cancer.

OTHER HORMONE THERAPY YOU MAY ENCOUNTER

Gonadotropin Releasing Hormone-antagonists (GnRH-antagonists)

This hormone is an estrogen blocker that interferes with the brain's release of the gonadotropin hormones (those hormones which stimulate the ovaries to produce estrogen.) (The term **antagonist** means *to work against*. Medically, it is a drug that blocks the action of a certain hormone.) These hormones are used to treat endometriosis since endometrial tissues thrive on estrogen. The side effects of the GnRH-antagonists are the same as in menopause, such as hot flashes, insomnia, depression, breast tenderness, vaginal dryness, reduced sex drive, and osteoporosis. These hormones probably should be not taken longer than 6 months and never when pregnant or if there is a chance of becoming pregnant.

Human Chorionic Gonadotropin (HCG)

HCG is a gonadotropin hormone produced in the placenta. HCG can be extracted from the urine of pregnant women and given by injection to treat some kinds of infertility. Synthetic HCG is used in the treatment of **recurrent miscarriage** and certain types of **female and male infertility**.

Menotropin

Menotropin is a gonadotropin which contains both FSH and LH. It is extracted from the urine of women past menopause to **treat female infertility** due to a failure to ovulate. As hormone therapy, menotropins may be used together with HCG. Side effects may include multiple pregnancies or abdominal pain. Menotropins also **help stimulate sperm production** in infertile men although it may cause male breast enlargement.

CAUTION
Contact your doctor, pharmacist or the manufacturer for information about benefits and side effects of these hormone replacements.

DRUGS THAT MAY CAUSE INTERACTIONS (These are just a few contraindications. Consult your doctor or the *Physicians' Desk Reference.*)

Barbiturates (sedatives) Decreases progesterone and estrogen effectiveness. Reduces blood platelets, causes bleeding. Hastens elimination of estrogen from body.
Corticosteroid drugs (prednisone, cortisone, hydrocortisone) Replaces natural hormones. Reduces production of prostaglandins. Suppresses the hormones naturally produced by the adrenal glands. Increases blood pressure. Affects menstrual cycles. Affects blood clot formation.
Tamoxifen (used to fight breast cancer) Decreases estrogenic effect by blocking estrogen receptors. Can cause hot flashes, vaginal bleeding and uterine overgrowth.
Tricyclic Antidepressants Affects blood pressure and heart rhythm. Can cause breast enlargement.
Warfarin Blood thinner. Estrogen decreases effectiveness of warfarin.

TERMS

You may encounter these terms about prescription and non-prescription products.

Conjugated means combined.

Extracted is when a substance is removed by pressing, distilling, pulling out, etc. For example, orange juice is extracted from an orange.

Synthetic is when separate parts are put together. Most drugs are synthetic because they are composed of separate components put together in a laboratory. Synthetic drugs can be prescription or non-prescription.

Natural is a term that is loosely used. As in the case of estrogen replacement, the mare's urine is a natural substance. However, the drug is categorized as a synthetic because the estrogen components from that urine have been "assembled" in a laboratory. A truly natural product is one that has not been altered chemically in any way; at least, not man-made or put together in a laboratory. Most herbal products are technically synthetic although their initial components are natural.

19
Herbal Hormones
Non-Prescription Hormone Remedies

The term herb or herbal is used to describe any plant used medicinally, whether leaf, stem, root or bark. Even though they are derived from natural products, these over-the-counter hormones are synthetic since they are combined or processed in a laboratory. (This, of course, would not apply to products consumed directly, such as soybeans, tea leaves, etc.) Just as with prescription hormone replacements, non-prescription hormones may carry the same benefits, side effects and risks as naturally-produced estrogen and progesterone. Some work better than others. And some carry such a high risk of adverse effects that they should be avoided. Let's look at some of the more common herbals.

DO THEY or DON'T THEY WORK?

Since most herbal products are not FDA tested and approved, there may not be proof of the health claims made by the manufacturer. So, do they work or don't they? That may just depend with whom you talk. One woman may swear by flaxseed whereas another woman will say it didn't help her at all. Without question, some of the products actually do what they say. For others, if the woman THINKS it's helping, then that's enough. You may be familiar with **placebos**. They are "dummy" drugs, usually sugar pills that have no medicinal benefit. But when given to people who THINK they are getting the real thing, they FEEL better. This may happen with some of these over-the-counter remedies. If you think they help and you feel better, than you've achieved your goal.

CAUTION
Just be careful of everything you put in your mouth. Don't assume that just because herbals are "natural" and non-prescription that they can be consumed willy-nilly. Don't take any pill or tea just because your neighbor does. Do your own research. Talk to your doctor. Be informed and safe.

PHYTO (Plant) ESTROGENS

Estrogens derived from plants are called **phyto-estrogens**. The active ingredients in most phytos are **isoflavones**. Since these are so chemically similar to estrogen, they are called plant estrogens. Some frequently mentioned phyto-estrogens are soy products, black cohosh, flaxseed, and dong quai.

These phyto-estrogens, particularly soy, came to light when it was realized many of these foods and herbs are included in the diet of women in Asia who have few menopausal symptoms. However, since Asian women have used them all their life, there is question whether adding them at the onset of menopause may be too late for a significant effect. (FYI: Asian women who adopt a Western diet will begin to experience symptoms associated with the Change of Life.)

Plant or herbal products seems to work best on mild menopausal symptoms like hot flashes and night sweats. It is not certain whether specific ones do or do not appear to increase the risk of endometrial or breast cancer. Some phytos appear to raise HDL (good) cholesterol which drops in menopause. There is discussion whether phytos help with osteoporosis.

Because they are **estrogenic**, the side effects of phyto-estrogens may be the same as with prescription hormone therapy. For example, with some synthetic estrogens, you may need a progesterone product to override the risks of uterine cancer. Side effects might include headache, insomnia (since many are stimulants), or bleeding (since many have blood-thinning characteristics.)

Herbal hormones, even those purchased without a prescription, can be as expensive as prescription drugs. Also, it is not advisable to mix both prescription and non-prescription hormone replacements. They may counteract each other. Worse, it would be like taking a double dose of estrogen and/or progesterone, which can be very serious.

NOTE TO VEGETARIANS or ANIMAL RIGHTS-ists

Most non-prescription estrogens are derived from plants, whereas most prescription estrogens are derived from the urine of pregnant mares, so many vegetarians and animal rights supporters may choose to use plant estrogens instead of a product from an animal source.

SOY

Soybeans come the closest to being like the body's natural estrogen production. Some sources of soy include tofu, soy milk, soybeans and roasted soy nuts. Soy proponents believe that soy products soothe hot flashes, eliminate vaginal dryness, reduce the risk of breast cancer, slow bone loss and help lower LDL (bad) cholesterol. Soy is often used as a substitute for red meat by vegetarians and those trying to lower their blood cholesterol.

BLACK COHOSH

Black Cohosh is derived from the buttercup family and was used by Native American Indian women to treat feminine problems. Black cohosh proponents believe this herb can help with hot flashes, night sweats and vaginal dryness. It may be that black cohosh reduces the secretion of the *Luteinizing Hormone* (LH). Minor side effects may include upset stomach, and a serious side effect may link black cohosh with uterine cancer as this herb is an estrogenic. There is another herb called *blue cohosh,* which is not the same as black cohosh but does claim benefits for menopausal complaints. (Read more about LH in Chapter 6.)

CHAMOMILE

Chamomile is most associated with having a calming, sedative effect. Menopausal claims are that it may reduce uterine cramps.

CHASTEBERRY *(Vitex) (Chaste tree)*

Chasteberry comes from the chaste tree (Vitex) and is usually associated with PMS. Proponents believe this herb reduces levels of *prolactin* which is associated with PMS. Chasteberry may relieve hot flashes and night sweats. Minor side effects may be rash, stomachache, or headache. Chasteberry has been used for centuries in monasteries to curb the sex drive in monks and is often known as "Monk's Pepper." (Read more about prolactin in Chapter 6.)

DONG QUAI (Dong Kwai) (Chinese Angelica)

Dong Quai is one of the most hotly debated herbs. Enthusiasts believe it relieves hot flashes. Non-enthusiasts believe it is not helpful. It is known to have blood-thinning characteristics and is a mild laxative. Dong Quai has long been used in China although in a combination with other herbs, and it's not certain which of the herbs provide symptom relief and which do not.

FLAXSEED

Ground flaxseed proponents believe this product from the flax plant may reduce the risk of breast cancer and lessen hot flashes and night sweats. A tablespoon or so is usually added at breakfast to oatmeal or cereal. (FYI: The seeds from the flax plant are used to make linseed oil, and the stem fibers can be spun into linen thread.)

GINSENG

Ginseng root has been used as an herbal remedy by the Chinese for many years. Ginseng proponents believe it may help reduce hot flashes and vaginal dryness. Ginseng is believed to be estrogenic and may stimulate endometrial growth and uterine bleeding. Another side effect of Ginseng may be breast tenderness. Ginseng is also used as an energy stimulant

LICORICE ROOT

Licorice root is from the licorice plant of the legume family and has long been used in herbal remedies and as a flavoring for black licorice candy. As a phyto-estrogen, it appears to contain high levels of estrogen-like compounds that affect the body like a weak dose of estrogen. Proponents believe it may relieve hot flashes and mood swings. Opponents believe it may actually induce hot flashes and other menopausal symptoms.

RED CLOVER

Red clover proponents believe this plant may help with hot flashes and vaginal dryness. It may contain blood-thinning characteristics.

PHYTO (Plant) PROGESTERONES

WILD YAMS *(Diosgenin)*

Just like prescription progesterone, over-the-counter progesterones are also derived from a compound in wild yams called *diosgenin.* Whereas drug manufacturers use only the molecule of progesterone separated from the rest of the diosgenin compound, herbal remedies may include both progesterone and unconverted diosgenin which remains in its original form as wild yam. This amount should be noted on the product to let you know the percentage of synthetic progesterone. For example, if a progesterone cream says 10% diosgenin, you are getting 90% of a progesterone and 10% of the wild yam extract that was not converted. Over-the-counter progesterone is most commonly found in cream form. Proponents believe this is the same as naturally produced progesterone. Opponents question whether this progesterone can actually be used by the body. (Wild yams are also purported to help with rheumatism and colic.)

WARNING

Non-prescription progestin should never be used alongside prescription progesterone.

20
Vitamin and Mineral Supplements

In an ideal world, we would get all our vitamins and minerals from the food we eat. But this isn't a perfect world. Fast food, frozen meals, and deli dishes from the grocery store probably aren't giving us all the nutrients we need. It's a rare woman who eats the correct portions from that perfect-food pyramid. So, it's a good idea to take a multiple vitamin and mineral supplement daily.

Unlike herbals, most vitamins and minerals have been studied over and over and have been proven to be vital for good health. For example, **Vitamin A** promotes healthy bones and healthy skin. The **B vitamins** interact with the chemicals in the body that break down and use carbohydrates, and they are essential for a healthy heart. **Vitamin C** is necessary for healthy bones and blood vessels. **Vitamin D** is vital for healthy bones and the proper absorption of calcium. **Vitamin E** benefits the skin and prevents premature aging. **Vitamin K** promotes blood clotting. This is, of course, just a BRIEF look at some vitamins. (Discussion about various minerals is found in Chapter 13.) For more information about the specific benefits and interactions of vitamins and minerals, talk to your doctor or research the internet. We will take just a minute, though, to look a little closer at **Vitamin E** and the **antioxidants,** and how they may be of special benefit to menopausal women.

VITAMIN E

Vitamin E is from the *tocopherol* family. The word comes from two Greek words with strong references to female fertility. *TOCO* (*childbirth*) and *PHER* (*to bear*). There is no question that Vitamin E is essential for overall good health. There are arguments on both sides of the fence whether Vitamin E actually affects fertility although many believe it helps with some menopausal symptoms such as hot flashes and headaches. Also, because Vitamin E works to disintegrate blood clots, it is certainly beneficial to everyone, especially women taking HRT. Finally, it is a fact that estrogen is a **Vitamin E antagonist** which means it neutralizes or counteracts Vitamin E, so it's a good idea to be sure this vitamin is a part of your daily vitamin regimen.

ANTIOXIDANTS

We also want to look at **antioxidants** and menopause. **Vitamins C, E,** and **A (beta carotene)** are antioxidants. They fight against oxidation which is the union of oxygen with any substance. (This is the same process that causes metals to rust and oils to become rancid.) Inside the body, oxidation causes free radicals which change the chemical structure in molecules and which are associated with cancer and other diseases. An antioxidant slows down the deterioration of cells which results when oxygen unites with fats and oils. In menopausal women, this is important because estrogen has already disrupted the overall chemical process, and especially the metabolism of fat which can create problems with cholesterol and arterial plaque. (see Chapter 12)

21
Seals of Approval
On Non-Prescription Products

You need to be aware that herbal products and dietary supplements purchased over the counter are not always studied and regulated like prescriptions which come under years of scrutiny by the Food and Drug Administration (FDA). There may be huge variations from product to product in the amount of "active ingredient" the product claims. In some cases, labeled amounts are one hundred percent accurate; in other cases, there may be much less or even much more of the product than specified on the bottle. In addition, you may find *labels* or *seals of approval*. Some of the certifying companies have been unfairly criticized for charging fees for testings and subsequent approval listings even though product testing can be multi-faceted and expensive. (Also, some of these companies are not-for-profit organizations.) Let's look at a few of these (in alphabetical order.)

ConsumerLab.com Its label indicates the product is contaminant free, properly dissolves in the stomach so that it is best utilized by the body, and that what is on the label is in the bottle. It also requires product consistency so that what is in one bottle is the same thing that is in them all. Started in 1999, ConsumerLab.com does not charge for all product testings but does charge if a company wants their product to have this specific seal.

BIOAVAILABILITY
is the technical term for a product properly dissolving in the stomach for best absorption in the body.

Good Housekeeping Institute Its label indicates that what is on a product label is actually in the bottle. GHI requires manufacturers to verify health claims on their products although GHI, itself, does only limited testing. Many companies want to advertise in *Good Housekeeping Magazine*, but they will only take advertisements from companies who can prove their product meets product evaluation standards. When these tests are passed, the product will receive the *Good Housekeeping Seal of Approval.* The Good Housekeeping Institute began in 1900. Supplements are just one category they test.

www.gh-atyourservice.com

NSF International Its label indicates the product is contaminant free and that what is on the label is in the bottle. This non-profit company started in 1944 as the National Sanitation Foundation and was dedicated to setting standards for the food service industry. Testing dietary supplements is just one of their categories. Others include bottled water, indoor air, and environmental issues. Most companies pay for NSF certification. www.nsf.org

USP (U.S.Pharmacopeia) Its label indicates the product is contaminant free, was produced under sanitary conditions, that what is on the label is actually in the bottle, and that the product will dissolve in the stomach fast enough to be of value to the body. USP has been setting standards for prescriptions and over-the-counter drugs since the 1820's. USP charges companies for its services and its seal. In the year 2000, USP created the Dietary Supplement Verification Program (DSVP) to meet the growing demand for over-the-counter dietary supplements.

www.usp.gov www.usp-dsvp.org

22
Diet and Exercise

Maintaining a healthy weight and keeping physically active is always important, and especially during the menopausal years. Because fat tissues convert into estrogen the hormones produced by the adrenal glands, it's important to not have too many fat cells. For example, the size of the breast increases as weight is gained. Since the breast is primarily fat, excess estrogen may "accumulate" in the breast. This can increase the risk of breast cancer.

Being physically active helps burn calories which prevents weight gain. This is especially important because, as we age, estrogen causes our metabolism to slow down, meaning that our bodies don't burn calories as fast as they used to. In fact, we usually need about 2/3 the calories as we did before menopause. However, all weight gain can't be attributed to menopause. As we age, we usually become less active which means weight gain is more likely.

Besides weight control, physical activity is a must for many conditions associated with menopause. By accelerating all movements throughout our system, physical exercise may decrease the exposure of the breast tissues and endometrial lining to circulating estrogen, which may lower the risk of cancer in these areas. This same acceleration helps our system to better process food, cutting down on constipation, heartburn, fluid retention and weight gain.

Weight-bearing exercises may reverse osteoporosis by building new bone. At the very least, they may stop bone loss. These include walking, jogging, and weight-lifting. Exercise also replenishes the **synovial fluid** that lubricates joints and prevents stiffness and muscle tension. Emotional tension can also be relieved because, when we exercise, **endorphins** are released that promote a "feel good" sensation. Besides making us feel better during the day, exercise greatly aids in sleep. And, of course, exercise maintains healthy lungs and heart, especially at a time when estrogen is a causing a loss of strength in all muscles, including the heart muscle.

We'd probably feel a lot better
if we would eat only the food
God provided for us. You'll notice there are
no cupcake trees or soda pop rivers.

23
Male Menopause

In most cases, men remain fertile most of their life. We've all heard stories about elderly men fathering children in their late 70's, sometimes even older. Unlike estrogen, testosterone does not fade out and go away, rendering a man infertile. However, there are two levels of testosterone. Within the "total" level is what is called "free" testosterone. Free testosterone is that part of the hormone that is not bound to a protein. So while the total level of testosterone may not decrease much as men age, the concentration of "free" testosterone may fall. This usually happens between the ages of 40 and 65 and may result in diminished sex drive, impotency, weight gain, and some loss of muscle and bone strength. No wonder they may get depressed and frustrated! Blood tests can be administered to check levels of both these testosterones but even if the free testosterone level is low, it's usually not necessary to resort to hormone replacement since the total testosterone is still being produced. Except in extreme cases, hormone replacement won't help much; and adding more could certainly cause problems. (Men should see their doctor for more information.)

When women are menopausal, it's because they have stopped having periods. Obviously, this can't be the case with men. Rather than a physiological matter, male "menopause" is more of a psychological issue. A more correct term would be **mid-life crisis.** In the same way it affects women, entering middle age puts men face to face with all their dreams and realities. Many of the goals and aspirations they had in their 20's probably haven't been met. They don't like the idea of getting old, but they can't avoid that reality. Their mirror may reflect gray hair, wrinkled skin, and even a pot belly. They are faced with their own mortality as they experience medical concerns or watch their own parents age and/or die. Like women, men may have just gone through 20 or more years of raising kids. Plus they are ever-influenced by the never-ending societal pressures of new cars, houses, and careers. For men and women alike, these issues have to be dealt with on a practical basis. Otherwise, depression, anxiety, and even serious physical concerns like heart attack and stroke may develop.

Men, be assured your wife loves you even if you HAVE gotten older and even if you haven't achieved all those dreams. You two have shared a LIFE together. When you look at your wife, you see beyond a few wrinkles or sprinkling of gray hairs. She loves you just the same way. Look with pride at how you have provided for your family, at the children you have raised, and at the glorious future you have ahead of you.

Be Thankful
For What You Have *and*
For Who You Are

24
Surviving the Change of Wife
Help for Husbands

Your Lassie has turned into a Pit Bull. Your Rock of Gibraltar has turned into Niagara Falls. Yep. The woman in your life has changed. It's called the *Change of Life.* Well, actually the medical term is **menopause**. But whatever it's called, it is going to change your life, too. Without going into a lot of medical jargon, we're going to explain to you what's going on in her body to cause the changes in her personality.

The hormones in her body are starting to get all out of whack. Her body used to put out a nice even amount of a hormone called estrogen. Estrogen is what makes her a woman. It's what makes her skin soft, gave her full breasts, and caused her to have monthly periods. If you have kids, they wouldn't be here without your wife's estrogen. But somewhere between the ages of 40 and 50, those hormones stopped coming in well-balanced amounts. There is either too much estrogen being produced, or not nearly enough. This is not a good thing.

This estrogen comes from a part of her body called an ovary. She has two of them. When she gets in her 40's, the ovaries start to shut down. HOWEVER, if your wife has had a surgery where both of her ovaries were removed, or if they have become diseased or damaged by something like chemotherapy or radiation, she will go through the Change of Life no matter what age she is.

The Change starts when your wife first starts noticing that her monthly periods aren't regular like they used to be. The doctors call the stage from when it first starts until when your wife actually stops having periods as the *pre-menopause* or *perimenopause*. Medically, the actual *menopause* is when a woman has had no periods for one year, but the real world lumps the entire process into the general term *menopause*.

Hopefully, your wife hasn't experienced the wild symptoms called PMS or pre-menstrual syndrome. But if she did, you know all about what can happen when hormones go wild. Anger. Tears. Irritability. Totally unpredictable behavior. Well, with the Change, you may be in for a lot of You-Ain't-Seen-Nothin'-Yet.

HOT FLASHES

The estrogen in her body is going to come on in big spurts and then back off just as quickly. This causes **hot flashes**. People laugh at hot flashes, but they're not funny to your wife. She is going to get very hot, then cool down quickly. This may happen many times a day. It usually doesn't have anything to do with the actual temperature in the room or outside. So don't be surprised when she turns up the a/c when you're already freezing or if she turns down the furnace just when you're getting toasty warm. And just when you're getting readjusted to the temperature, she'll jump up and change the thermostat again. Believe me, this is bothering her a lot more than it is bothering you. Watch out when she utters the words made famous by menopausal women, "Is it hot in here? Or is it just me?"

NIGHT SWEATS

These hot flashes are also going to make it really hard for her to sleep. When they happen at night, they're called **night sweats**. When a hot flash hits at night, the heat gets trapped in your wife's pajamas and the blankets she's wrapped up in. There's no place for this heat to escape, so her body produces lots of sweat in an attempt to cool down. She may awaken drenched in her own sweat. And this might happen many times during the night. If you wake up to find that she has relocated to the spare bedroom or onto the sofa, don't be offended. She's just desperate for a cool place to sleep. So if she temporarily needs to leave your bed, don't take it personally. In fact, you may find that you'll sleep better, too, if she's not there. It's pretty hard to get a good night's sleep when your mate is fanning the covers all night long!

SEX

Another thing that's going to affect you directly as a man concerns sex. Before menopause came long, estrogen created a favorable environment which made it easy for the two of you to have sex. But now estrogen has caused her tissues to dry out. So, when you first get started in sex, she may experience some pain due to the dryness. There are products either of you can use that will solve most of this problem. Take it slow and easy.

On the other hand, many women find that they enjoy sex a lot more now at this menopausal time. When your wife was still having normal periods, there was always a chance she might get pregnant, whether she wanted to or not. Once her periods stop, that will not be a worry. Also, since her periods will soon be ending, there won't be any off-limit days for sex. You two may find that sex is more enjoyable than ever.

EMOTIONS

Speaking of getting pregnant, permanently losing their ability to have children can be pretty **upsetting** for some women. This was a big part of your wife's woman-ness, and she may actually need time to mourn this loss of fertility. The forever-gone chance to bear children can be especially hard on a woman who never had kids but wanted them. It can be equally hard on women who did become mothers, because they may be losing their child-bearing abilities at the same time their kids are growing up and leaving home. For a while, the **empty-nest syndrome** can be pretty sad for moms (and dads.)

Sadness may be only one of a bunch of emotions your wife will be working through. Estrogen fluctuations are going to make her moods swing wildly. Of course, this is going to affect you. If she starts crying for no reason, it's probably NOT because of something you did. She can't help the feeling; it just washes over her with no warning. She may also get cranky or downright mean. This is not intentional. In addition to female hormones, your wife's body also puts out a small amount of some male hormones. These help in ways like giving her muscles strength. Up until now, these male hormones have been kept minimized by the over-powering amount of female hormones. But when estrogen (the female hormone) starts to fade out, some of the male hormones come to the fore-front. These same male hormones that have given YOU big, bulky muscles, a deep voice, and whiskers on your face are also responsible for aggressive personality traits. This aggression is what's coming out in your wife now. But rest assured that this is only temporary and she will soon return to her normal personality. The emotional roller coaster ride does, eventually, end.

MEMORY

Your wife may also have all kinds of trouble remembering things because estrogen affects **memory**, too. So if she asks you a question several times, or can't remember something you just said, try to be patient. Don't automatically think that she's getting Alzheimer's disease. Although there may be a connection with estrogen loss and eventually developing Alzheimer's, that's probably not the problem here. And don't think that she's just not paying attention. You're not going to help anything if you give a quick, "I just told you that. Aren't you listening?" You do that during menopause, and you may have a wife dissolve in tears or get terribly angry!

HOW LONG IS THIS GOING TO LAST?

Now don't panic, but this roller coaster ride can last ten years or more. It's not a quick, *let's get it over with* kind of deal. The first five or six years will be the worst for the hot flashes and mood changes. And don't think that it's all over when your wife finally stops having periods. It's not. The hot flashes and all the rest of it can go on many years more because the estrogen doesn't all go away at once. So please don't ask, "Isn't it about time for this thing to be over?"

IS THERE SOME KIND OF PILL TO STOP THIS?

By now, you're asking if there is some kind of pill she can take to make it go away. The answer is, kind of. Her doctor will offer some pills called Hormone Replacement Therapy (HRT). A long time ago, doctors learned that they can take the urine from pregnant horses (mares), extract the estrogen from it, and give it to women in the form of pills, creams or even a patch.

This medication will get rid of the hot flashes, vaginal dryness and moodiness. However, this does not come without a price. Adding the estrogen can also put your wife at a high risk for developing breast cancer or cancer of the uterus. The doctors can prescribe another hormone called progesterone that your wife's body also used to make. This can offset the risk of the uterine cancer, but there is still the breast cancer issue. And there are many other medical problems linked to both estrogen and progesterone hormone replacement therapy. So your wife has a big decision to make. Will solving one problem now cause another problem later?

Although you can make suggestions, you can't make the final medical decisions for your wife. What you CAN do, is be loving. This is a medical issue and should be treated as such. Treat her with the same tenderness and attention you would give her if she had the flu or a serious illness. Don't be patronizing or overly mushy, but remember that this is the woman who has always taken care of everyone else when they were down and out. You do the same for her now. She will love you for it!

Remember:
You pledged through good times AND bad times.

25
Meno Moms
For the kids

If it seems that your mom is acting kind of weird, that she's changed from the mom you're used to, it's because she has. It's what is called the **Change of Life**. There are chemicals inside her body that are changing. They are going to make her sad so that she'll cry for no reason. They may even make her mad for no reason. (She's going to try to not take this out on you.) They are also going to make her hot, and then cold, and then hot and cold again. Over and over. This will happen during the day and also at night. That's why you might see her changing the thermostat a lot.

You know how sometimes you don't feel really good, but you're not sick enough to go to bed? You might still go to school or go ahead and play with your friends. Well, your mom is feeling kind of like that now. She'll still be able to take care of you. She'll still do everything she always did. She's just going to feel kind of weird for a while. Your mom will soon be back to her regular self. Hang in there! And be sure to ask your mom if you have any more questions about why she has turned into Meno Mom.

TOP TEN REASONS

TOP TEN REASONS MENOPAUSE IS GOOD

10. Get to read the *Menopause Survival Guide*
9. No Periods
8. No chance of getting pregnant
7. No Periods
6. Good excuse for not remembering anything
5. Great conversation starter with any woman
4. No Periods
3. No Periods
2. No Periods
1. NO PERIODS!!!!

TOP TEN REASONS MENOPAUSE IS BAD

10. Creaky bones
9. Can't remember anything
8. No chance of getting pregnant
7. Too many technical terms
6. Tearful moods
5. Cranky moods
4. Down-right mean moods
3. Facial hair
2. Hot flashes
1. Night sweats

GLOSSARY

ADRENAL GLAND Either of a pair of endocrine organs, lying immediately above the kidney, which produce a variety of steroid hormones.

AMENORRHEA Absence of menstruation.

ANABOLIC METABOLISM Chemical process that builds up a substance for use.

ANDROGEN HORMONES A group of sex hormones that cause the development of male characteristics such as the growth of facial hair, voice deepening, and an increase in muscle bulk. Production of the androgen hormones are controlled by the pituitary gland. The most active and potent androgens are produced by the testes (male). Small amounts are secreted by the ovaries until menopause. Although the adrenal glands produce androgens in both the males and females, they are usually less active and rarely have a significant masculinizing effect. An imbalance of the androgen hormones in females can occasionally cause ovarian tumors and an increase in body hair. From the root *ANDRO* (*man*) + *GEN* (*something that produces or is produced).*

ARTERIOSCLEROSIS A group of disorders that causes thickening and loss of elasticity of artery walls. Atherosclerosis is the most common type of arteriosclerosis.

ATHEROSCLEROSIS A thickening and loss of elasticity of the walls of the arteries. The most common type of arteriosclerosis.

ATROPHY A wasting away of a body tissue or organ due to not being nourished.

AUTONOMIC NERVOUS SYSTEM The part of the nervous system that controls the involuntary, automatic activities of organs, blood vessels, glands, and other tissues. These activities cannot be controlled consciously by the brain but are automatically carried out by the body.

AXILLARY Pertaining to the underarm area. Often referenced when a mastectomy has been performed as this is the location of many lymph nodes.

BENIGN Mild or not growing. When referring to cancer, this means that a tumor will not spread to another part of the body.

CAPILLARY Very tiny, narrow blood vessels.

CAROTENE A substance found in certain colored plants and vegetables that is converted by the body into Vitamin A.

CAROTENOID A yellow or red plant or animal pigment (coloring agent). Connected with carotene, a substance the body turns into Vitamin A.

CATABOLIC METABOLISM Chemical process that breaks down a substance for use.

CELE Suffix meaning *rupture* or *swelling.*

CLIMACTERIC (*Rung of a ladder*) (*Climax*) A period in the life of a person when an important physiological change occurs, especially referring to the time of menopause.

CONJUGATED Combined.

CORPUS (*Body*) The main part of an organ. A mass of tissue with a specialized function.

CORPUS LUTEUM A mass of yellow tissue formed in the ovary by a ruptured follicle that has discharged its egg; if the egg is fertilized, this tissue secretes the hormone progesterone that is needed to maintain a pregnancy. *CORPUS* (*body*) + *LUTEUM* (*yellow*)

CORTICOSTEROID HORMONES Group of hormones produced by the adrenal glands that control the body's use of nutrients and the excretion of salts and water in the urine.

CYSTOCELE Surgery to reposition front vaginal wall. Condition caused by the bladder pushing against a weakened vaginal wall. May cause the urethra to be displaced.

DEEP-VEIN THROMBOSIS Clotting of blood within the deep-lying veins, usually in the legs, generally caused by a combination of sluggish blood flow through one part of the body and some factor that increases the tendency of the blood to clot. Often in people who have been immobilized for a great length of time.

DIOSGENIN A compound found in wild yams that contains a molecule of progesterone that can be converted to a progesterone similar to what the body makes. Conversion can only be done in a lab. Then this form of progesterone is added to a product. On a product label, *diosgenin* denotes the amount of the wild yam that was NOT converted to progesterone.

DOWAGER A widow with some valuable property inherited from her dead husband. Also an elderly woman of wealth and dignity. This wealth was the *dowry* or gift she would bring into another marriage.

DYSMENORRHEA Painful periods. Term for cramps associated with menstrual periods. *DYS* is a prefix for *bad.*

ECTOMY A suffix meaning *to cut out.* Example: a tonsillectomy is the removal of the tonsils.

EGG Same as *ovum.* The reproductive cell produced by the female in the ovary.

EMBOLISM The blockage of an artery by a clump of material traveling in the bloodstream. The particle causing the blockage is called an *embolus* and may be a blood clot (most common), a bubble of air or gas, a piece of tissue or tumor, a clump of bacteria, bone marrow, cholesterol or fat. Travels in the bloodstream where it eventually causes an arterial obstruction.

ENDOCRINE Any gland producing one or more internal secretions that are introduced directly into the bloodstream and carried to other parts of the body whose functions they regulate or control.

ENDOMETRIAL HYPERPLASIA An overgrowth of the uterine lining due to too much estrogen and not enough (or no) progesterone. Can be a forerunner of cancer.

ENDOMETRIUM The inner lining of the uterus. (see *Uterine Lining*) It is the endometrium that is shed monthly if there is no fertilized egg.

EQUINE Having to do with horses.

ESTRADIOL An estrogen produced by the ovaries. Converted into estrone and estriol. Also produced synthetically for HRT.

ESTRIOL An estrogen converted from estradiol.

ESTROGEN Any of several female sex hormones. Necessary for female reproductive system and female characteristics. From the suffix *GEN (something that produces or is produced)* and *ESTROUS.*

ESTRONE An estrogen converted from estradiol before onset of menopause. After menopause, estrone is the estrogen converted in fat cells from hormones released by adrenal glands. Also produced synthetically for HRT.

ESTROUS CYCLE A regular female reproductive cycle that is under hormonal control. Includes a period of heightened libido (sex drive), followed by ovulation and then complex changes of the uterine lining.

ESTRUS In the animal kingdom, when a female animal will accept mating with the male. From the root word *frenzy*. Known as when the female animal is *in heat.*

EXTRACTION To draw out or remove by pressing, distilling, etc. Example: orange juice is extracted from an orange.

FIBROIDS Abnormal growths that may occur inside or outside the walls of the uterus. They are almost always benign although they may cause heavy bleeding and discomfort. (see *Myoma*)

FLUSH A sudden feeling of great heat. Caused by the capillaries in the skin suddenly opening which causes a rush of blood intended to cool the body by sweating. Also commonly called "flash."

FOLLICLE A small sac, cavity, or gland for excretion or secretion.

FOLLICLE STIMULATING HORMONE (FSH) Secreted by the pituitary gland, a hormone which stimulates the development of eggs (ova) in the female and the development of testicular function in the male.

FOLLICULAR STAGE Also called *Proliferative Stage.* A stage during the menstrual cycle when an egg is being developed within a follicle within an ovary.

GINGIVITIS An inflammation of the gums caused by plaque build-up.

GONAD An organ in animals that produces reproductive cells, especially an *ovary* or the *testes.*

GONADOTROPIN HORMONE A hormone which supports and stimulates the function and growth of the gonads (ovaries or testes). From the root *GONAD* (*ovaries or testes*) + *TROPIN* (*stimulant*)

HEART ATTACK Damage to part of the heart due to impaired blood supply to the heart. May result in death.

HORMONE From the Greek word meaning *to stimulate.* A substance formed in some organ of the body, as the adrenal glands, the pituitary, etc., and carried by a body fluid to another organ or tissue, where it has a specific effect.

HOT FLASH Same as *flush.*

HYPOTHALAMUS A part of the brain near the pituitary gland that is a kind of control center for hormone messengers

HYSTERECTOMY The surgical removal of all or part of the uterus.

ISOFLAVONES Plant estrogens.

LUTEAL PHASE Also called the *secretory phase*. Refers to the second half of the menstrual cycle when the corpus luteum secretes progesterone.

LUTEIN A yellow carotenoid pigment found in green leafy vegetables, egg yolks, and in certain hormones. Lutein (*LOO-teen*) is a carotenoid found in vegetables and fruits. Acts as an antioxidant, protecting cells against the damaging effects of free radicals.

LUTEINIZING Stimulating the production of the corpus luteum.

LUTEINIZING HORMONE A hormone, secreted by the pituitary gland, which stimulates ovulation and the development of the corpus luteum for its subsequent secretion of progesterone, in females. Also stimulates the development of tissues in the testes and the secretion of testosterone in the testes of men.

LUTEINIZING HORMONE-RELEASING HORMONES Luteinizing hormone-releasing hormones stimulate the release of gonadotropin hormones from the pituitary gland. Gonadotropin hormones, in turn, control the production of the estrogen hormones and the androgen hormones. These control the level of cell activity in the organs stimulated by the sex hormones, such as the uterus, breasts, ovaries, testes, and prostate gland. A reduction in these hormones may cause headache, nausea, hot flashes, vaginal dryness, and irregular periods.

MALIGNANT Growing and becoming worse. When referring to a cancer, this means that a tumor will, or has, spread to another part of the body.

MAMMOGRAMS An important diagnostic procedure in the detection of breast abnormalities.

MELANOCYTE-STIMULATING HORMONE (MSH) Hormone secreted by the pituitary gland that acts on the skin to produce skin pigmentation (melanin).

MENARCHE (*men ARE key*) A girl's first menstrual period.

MENOPAUSE *MENO* (*month, moon*) + *PAUSE* (*to cause to stop*) The permanent cessation of menstruation, normally between the ages of 40 and 50. Also known as the C*hange of Life* or the *female climacteric.*

MENORRHAGIA Excessive bleeding during the menstrual period. Due to hormone imbalance, fibroids, polyps, and other causes.

MENSES Monthly menstrual periods. Plural of *mensis.*

METASTASIS When a malignant cancer spreads from an initial area to another place in the body.

METRORRHAGIA Extremes in the menstrual cycle such as intervals between periods, length of time bleeding occurs, and the amount of blood expelled.

MNEMONIC (*nee MON ick*) To help to remember.

MYO Prefix for *muscle.*

MYOCARDIAL INFARCTION Heart attack.

MYOMA Non-cancerous tumor of muscle.

MYOMECTOMY Surgery to remove a myoma. Type of surgery to remove fibroid tumor from uterine wall.

NATURAL Substance that is produced or existing in nature and not manufactured or artificial.

OLIGOMENORRHEA Light or few menstrual periods.

OOPHORECTOMY The surgical removal of one (unilateral) or both (bilateral) ovaries. (*oophor* sounds like *two-fer*)

OSTEOPOROSIS *OSTEO* (*bone*) + *POROSIS* (*porous)* A bone disease characterized by a reduction in bone density accompanied by increasing porosity and brittleness.

OVA Plural of *ovum*. Eggs.

OVARY Either of the pair of female reproductive glands producing eggs and sex hormones. Each ovary consists of glandular cells and egg-producing follicles. After ovulation, each follicle forms a corpus luteum. Each ovary contains numerous cavities called follicles in which egg cells develop. Ovaries are responsible for most of the body's estrogen and progesterone production.

OVUM (*Egg*) The reproductive cell produced by the female. A mature female germ cell which, after fertilization, develops into a new member of the same species. (The fertilized egg is an *embryo*.)

PHYTO-ESTROGEN *PHYTO* (*plant*) An estrogen derived from a plant basis.

PITUITARY GLAND A small, oval endocrine gland at the base of the brain that secretes hormones influencing body growth, metabolism, the activity of other endocrine glands, etc.

PLAQUE (Arterial) Refers to raised spots of fat, cholesterol, calcium, etc. that may accumulate and narrow or block arteries.

PLAQUE (Dental) A sticky accumulation of food particles, saliva, and bacteria that are deposited on the teeth near the gumline.

POLYMENORRHEA Menstrual periods come too often (less than 22 days between cycles.)

PROGESTERONE A steroid (sex) hormone secreted by the corpus luteum, active in preparing the uterus for the reception and development of the fertilized egg and the mammary glands for milk secretion. From the root words *PRO* (*promoting*) +*Gestation* + *Sterol.*

PROGESTIN Another name for a progesterone hormone or synthetic progesterone drug.

PROLACTIN A hormone secreted by the pituitary gland that stimulates milk production after childbirth. From the root words *PRO* (*promoting* or *in favor of*) and *LACTATE.*

PROLAPSE A displacement of part or all of an organ from its normal position.

PROLIFERATIVE STAGE Also called the follicular stage. A phase during the menstrual cycle when the egg is being developed within an ovarian follicle. *PRO* (*favorable for*) + *LIFE* (life, fertility)

PROSTAGLANDINS A broad term for a group of fatty acids that is made naturally in the body and that acts similarly to hormones. Occurs in many different body tissues including the semen, uterus, brain and kidneys. Effects include protecting the stomach lining from ulcers, stimulating uterine contractions during childbirth, and reducing the stickiness of blood platelets. A change in prostaglandins can affect blood clotting.

PULMONARY EMBOLISM (PE) An obstruction of the pulmonary artery or one of its branches in the lung by an embolus, usually a blood clot that originated in a vein in the leg or pelvis as a complication of deep-vein thrombosis. If the embolus is large enough to block the main pulmonary artery leading from the heart to the lungs, or if there are many clots, the condition may be life threatening. PE is responsible for tens of thousands of deaths in the U.S. each year. PE is usually the result of a fragment from a deep-vein thrombosis (a blood clot formed deep in a vein) breaking off and being carried via the heart to block an artery supplying the lungs.

RECTOCELE Surgery to reposition back vaginal wall. Condition is caused by rectum pushing against the weakened vaginal wall.

SECRETORY PHASE Also called the *luteal phase*. Refers to the second half of the menstrual cycle when the corpus luteum secretes progesterone.

SMOOTH MUSCLE One of three types of muscles. *Skeletal* muscles are those we can voluntarily control. *Cardiac* muscles are found only in the heart. *Smooth* muscles are those over which we have no conscious control but which respond to the nerve supply from the autonomic nervous system and which are affected by changes in hormones, oxygen levels, etc.

STATINS Drugs used to reduce cholesterol levels and prevent heart disease.

STEROID Any of a group of compounds including the sterols, bile acids, sex hormones, etc.

STEROLS (Such as cholesterol) Have a variety of functions within the body, often being converted by chemical actions into hormones or vitamins.

STRIA Stretch marks.

STROKE Damage to part of the brain due to interruption of blood supply.

SYNOVIAL FLUID A clear, sticky lubricant secreted by the membranes of movable joints. Liquid resembles egg whites.

SYNTHETIC *Put together.* When separate components are put together to form one product.

TESTES Plural of *testis*. The testicles.

TESTOSTERONE Male steroid (sex) hormone. From the root *TEST* (*testes*) + *STER* (*sterol*).

TETANY Involuntary spasms, often in the face around the lips, eyes or cheeks. Due to many causes, but for menopausal women usually due to anxiety. Twitches. (Not the same as *tics* which are usually the result of a psychological condition.)

TRANSIENT-ISCHEMIC ATTACK (TIA) Also called mini-stroke. Stroke symptoms that last for less than 24 hours and are followed by a full recovery. Usually only lasts for minutes. A warning sign that the brain is receiving an insufficient blood supply.

TROPIN A suffix meaning *to stimulate.* Example, a gonadotropin hormone stimulates the gonads.

URETHROCELE Surgery to reposition weakened front vaginal wall. May cause urethra to be displaced.

USP U.S. Pharmacopoeia.

UTERINE LINING Also called the *endometrium.* The inner lining of the uterus which receives the fertilized egg. The egg is nourished through the blood vessels in the lining. It is the uterine lining that is shed monthly if there is no fertilized egg.

UTERUS A thick-walled organ about 3 inches long where the fertilized egg grows into a baby.

VASO *Vessel.*

VASOCONSTRICTION Vessels narrow to reduce blood flow.

VASODILATATION Vessels widen to increase blood flow.

VASOMOTOR Regulates size of blood vessels by making them constrict and dilate. *VASO* (*vessel*) + *MOTOR* (*move*)

Sources and Websites to Check out

- American Cancer Society
  www.cancer.org
- American Heart Association
  www.americanheart.org
- American Medical Association
  www.ama-assn.org
- American Stroke
  www.strokeassociation.org
- Center for Disease Control
  www.cdc.gov
- Food and Drug Administration
  www.fda.gov
- National Cancer Institute
  www.nci.nih.gov
- National Institute for Health
  www.nih.gov
- National Osteoporosis Foundation
  www.nof.gov www.osteo.org
- Physicians' Desk Reference
  www.pdr.net
- Premature Ovarian Failure
  www.pofsupport.org

Contact Us

We would love to hear from you. Maybe you'd like to share how you've survived menopause. Or perhaps you have a childhood remembrance about "becoming a woman." Here's how to contact us.

Menopause Survival Guide
P. O. Box 28114
Kansas City, MO 64188-0114

E-mail:
SurviveMenopause@aol.com

Or visit us at
www.MenopauseSurvivalGuide.com

(None of your personal information, including your e-mail, will ever be sold or shared with any group.)

Thanks for reading the
Menopause Survival Guide.
God Bless You!

ORDER FORM

Here's how to share the *Menopause Survival Guide* with your family and friends.

PLEASE Send me __________ copies of the ***Menopause Survival Guide*** at $12.00 each. (U.S.)

Missouri residents add 6.9% sales tax. (82¢ per book)
U.S. residents add $2.00 shipping for each book.
Int'l Shipping: CAN $3.00, UK 6.00, AU $6.50

Name____

Organization (if applicable)__________________________

Address____

City/State/Zip_______________________________________

Phone____________________E-Mail___________________

To Purchase By Check or Money Order:
Please make checks payable to Oakview Press.
Mail to:
Oakview Press
P. O. Box 28114
Kansas City, MO 64188-0114
(Please attach a completed copy of this order form with your payment.)

To Purchase By Credit/Debit Card Online:
Visit us at:
www.MenopauseSurvivalGuide.com

www.MenopauseSurvivalGuide.com